Techniques of Hypnotic Induction

George Gafner

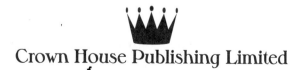

Crown House Publishing Limited

www.crownhouse.co.uk
www.crownhousepublishing.com

First published by

Crown House Publishing Ltd
Crown Buildings, Bancyfelin, Carmarthen, Wales, SA33 5ND, UK
www.crownhouse.co.uk

and

Crown House Publishing Company LLC
6 Trowbridge Drive, Suite 5, Bethel, CT 06801-2858, USA
www.crownhousepublishing.com

British Library Cataloguing-in-Publication Data
A catalogue entry for this book is available
from the British Library.

ISBN 978-184590292-6

LCCN 2009936670

Printed in the USA

To Sonja Benson and Matt Weyer

Acknowledgements

I would like to thank Susan Kelly Becker, Sonja Benson, Stephen Lankton, Dorothy Stoops and Michael Yapko for kindly agreeing to read the manuscript.

Contents

1. Introduction

Introduction

Let's say you've begun a long anticipated vacation and your final destination is Pleasure Island. This island represents the therapy phase of hypnotherapy. But first you have to *get* to the island. You board a cruise ship to take you to the island. This brief journey on the ship is the hypnotic induction.

The therapy phase of the process may consist of a story, an age regression, or any other myriad techniques (see Appendix I). But first you must successfully induce trance so that your client is prepared for what follows. That's what this book is about, the cruise ship, or induction. If your client's goal is simply relaxation, or a brief respite from the stress of everyday life, then one of the inductions in this book may be all you'll need for the session, both the cruise ship and island wrapped into one.

This book contains both directive inductions as well as ones that are indirect. The directive inductions are guided imagery experiences that invite clients to imagine immersing themselves in a structured experience, for example, walking down a path in the forest and participating in one image and then another. Guided imagery inductions are good for people who require structure, especially structures that contain realizable steps, one thing leading to another, like links in a chain, where a positive albeit unexpected outcome is built into the experience.

Other clients, though, appreciate less structure. Some people may be wary of hypnosis, or resistant to letting go. They do not like to be told what to feel, or they may have difficulty experiencing hypnotic phenomena, such as time distortion or amnesia. These clients may not like guided imagery inductions, much less an authoritarian approach such as, "Beginning now, I want you to develop a heaviness in your right hand ... that's right, make that hand as heavy as lead so that you can't lift it even an inch off your lap ..." Instead, I employ story inductions with these folks, as they tend to appreciate a permissive and indirect approach, one that permits them to experience any variety of hypnotic phenomena of their choosing. For most people who want to experience trance, I reach first for a story induction. The main thing about any induction is that the client *experience* something. Their experiencing catalepsy, dissociation, numbness or tingling in the extremities, or any other hypnotic phenomena, ratifies trance. They can then say, "Yes, indeed, I *experienced* something."

In both types of inductions I employ metaphor that strongly targets the unconscious, for it is in the unconscious where change begins. With story inductions, trance occurs when you read your client a story about *someone else* who develops interesting sensations in her body. Easy, non-threatening, and failsafe. Such a metaphorical approach gets in underneath the radar and cannot be defended against. So, for example, in the Glen Canyon induction (see Chapter 3), the client listens to a story about people taking a journey down the Colorado River. The people in the story experience dissociation, time distortion, and many other hypnotic phenomena, and trance is induced because the listener automatically self-references these phenomena. When clients don't respond to a story or guided imagery induction, I usually reach for a confusional induction. I have included two of these inductions for those clients whose unconscious resistance does not permit them to let go (see Chapter 6).

I have written four previous books on clinical hypnosis and conducted sessions with thousands of clients over thirty years as a therapist. I employ inductions ad lib but because I can't remember every induction – or story – I have come to rely on reading scripts. Our reading to clients becomes a natural part of the session. They readily expect and appreciate the caring and intimacy inherent in a carefully crafted and well read induction.

In addition to notes for practice, a glossary, and an appendix on techniques to choose from once trance is induced, along with a chapter on finding your hypnotic voice, this book features call-outs in some of the chapters. At conferences many people have told me they learn much from this device in which, say, "*she lost track of time*" is italicized in the text and next to it *time distortion* appears in the margin, thus explaining the principle or technique. In the notes for practice I try to anticipate the learning needs of the clinician. As such, I am especially interested in the personal growth and development of the therapist.

These inductions have been successfully employed with clients in the mental health clinic of the Veterans Affairs Health Care System in Tucson, Arizona. These are clients with personality disorders, medical problems, and a wide range of Axis I disorders including schizophrenia and substance use disorders, as well as mood and anxiety disorders. These are ready-made inductions for individuals or groups in your office or hospital practice. Others use these inductions in educational or wellness settings, or in practices where meditation, guided imagery, or relaxation techniques are customarily employed.

It is with privilege and pleasure that I offer you *Techniques of Hypnotic Induction*. Doing hypnotherapy is a gratifying – and sometimes challenging! – clinical activity. I am truly pleased that you have chosen this book to augment your professional practice.

2. Getting Started

Getting Started

What is hypnosis?

In 2005 the American Psychological Association (APA) adopted a new definition of hypnosis: "Hypnosis typically involves an introduction to the procedure during which the subject is told that suggestions for imaginative experiences will be presented" (Green et al., 2005: 104). Doesn't that have the clarity of a mud puddle and sound like it was written by company attorneys? Not something you want to tell clients if they ask you to define hypnosis. The above definition goes on to narrowly limit and obfuscate, along with reinforcing the negative stereotype of the client as a passive recipient instead of one who is an interactive participant in a cooperative venture (Yapko, 2005–2006).

That's why I prefer the APA's 1993 definition: "A procedure wherein changes in sensations, perceptions, thoughts, feelings, or behavior are suggested" (Gafner, 2004), something I include in a handout that I send to clients before the initial session. People also may have heard the following as defin itions: a narrowing of conscious attention, guided daydream ing, controlled dissociation, believed-in imagination, or myr iad other terms, and if they ask me if any of those are hypnosis, I say, "You bet." If they ask if guided imagery and meditation are hypnosis I say, "Yes, they are very similar to hypnosis," as they certainly could fall into the two APA definitions. Progres sive muscle relaxation (PMR), though, a commonly practiced procedure to relax the body, is not hypnosis, but if you throw in imagery, a story, or any other metaphorical suggestions, it starts to look like hypnosis. My general rule of thumb is this: it's hypnosis if you call it hypnosis.

I deeply respect any opinion by Michael D. Yapko, a clin ical psychologist in California who is regarded as one of the brightest and most articulate spokesmen in our field. He has a different take on this. He believes that hypnosis will not ad vance if we back off on definition. He believes that parallel procedures like meditation share *hypnotic qualities* with hyp nosis, but could never achieve full-blown hypnotic phenom ena such as an anesthesia that would withstand undergoing surgery. He believes that only with hypnosis can a client ex perience "substantial degrees of dissociation and automaticity of responses." He prefers to put the emphasis on the person's *experiencing* hypnosis and to this end he simply launches into his trademark permissive, hypnotic patter and leaves it up to clients whether or not they feel "hypnotized." Furthermore, he strongly opposes the policy of "giving people a mini-lec ture on misconceptions about hypnosis and then having them sign a waiver" (personal communication, 2009).

Negative stereotypes

In your practice you may not have a choice on policy matters such as waivers, as negative fears and preconceived notions may prevail. Many of us who practice hypnosis recognize that it is not only akin to other modalities but that it is also a modality predated thousands of years by ancient storytellers, medicine men, and religious healers, and connected as well to conveyances of suggestion in story, movie, and song whose metaphors reverberate in the unconscious mind. However, many people, including some mental health professionals, if asked about hypnosis, won't contemplate the exquisite legacy of human experience. Instead, their minds will turn to awe and mystery, or to heedless mind control, or "planted" memories to be recovered later, or hypnotized people on stage at a comedy club doing outrageous things. The awe or mystery of hypnosis may draw clients – and therapists – to it, just as the perception of mind control will repel others. Meditation and guided imagery don't have this potency and mystery and, as Dr. Yapko points out, we're not likely to see surgeries done where meditation is the sole anesthetic. However, meditation and guided imagery also don't carry the baggage of hypnosis. Two sides of the same coin: mystery and potency on one side, mind control on the other. I don't think you can have one without the other. When you practice hypnosis this legacy will likely come into play. You don't need a mini-lecture, but you can anticipate negative stereotypes by asking clients about preconceived notions, and clear the air during the first session. People often say things like, "I saw a stage hypnotist on TV. Is that hypnosis?" And I say, "Yes, and those guys are darn good, but let's get this clear: that's hypnosis for entertainment, this is hypnosis for helping people with a problem."

I'll always remember a man at Arizona Veterans Affairs who got referred for the hypnosis gastrointestinal study. Right off that man told me, "Your intentions to help me may be good, but in your background, even generations ago, there may have been a satanic person, and that person may be influencing you today." That guy wasn't psychotic; he was an educated, high functioning man who simply harbored a bizarre notion. The second those words came out of his mouth I sent him packing. In general, I believe, strong religiosity of any persuasion may be a contraindication to hypnosis. I typically do no hypnosis during the first session so I can dig into three important areas: negative stereotypes, the "magic bullet," and control issues. The times I've failed to do so I regretted it later.

The magic bullet

It always starts with good intentions – on our part as well as the client's. Of course we're eager to help, that's why we got into this business in the first place. But both client and therapist always need to look out for the magic bullet. Magic bullet, silver bullet, or unarticulated unrealistic expectations – you want to see if it's operating right from the start. It isn't always easy to ferret out and often doesn't rear its head until you've seen the person several times. The blatant examples are easy: "I want you to hypnotize me so I'll lose my desire for food and lose 100 pounds," or similar desires for tobacco and other substances. Be brief but respectful and then show them the door. You want to spend your time on people who can be helped. Your colleagues may send you their treatment failures for hypnosis. You hear from a colleague, "I have this woman who has failed six different SSRIs and various combinations of meds," or "He's been to every CBT and mindfulness group we offer." Appreciate the good intentions but listen for the report of the gun – a magic bullet is coming at you. One time a psychiatrist referred me one of his patients so I could help the guy with his headaches that were caused by the antidepressant Effexor. The doctor's intentions were good; Effexor was helping a lot except for those darn headaches. To be a good sport I saw the person a couple of times. He didn't respond and I sent him back to his doctor. Again, magic bullet.

Issues of control and intimacy

Here, we're not talking about trust. Clients will readily trust once you explain what you're doing and once they begin to relax and experience something positive. A separate issue, a major one, is control. This occurs to some extent in all clients new to hypnosis and it is vital that you monitor control issues, especially early in therapy.

First of all, those who are paranoid or highly anxious about your reading their mind or implanting something untoward in their unconscious, they won't show up in the first place. I'm talking about other clients who, for very good reasons, may think you're reading their mind because of your adept clinical skills. For example, during some phase of the process you notice eye flutter beneath closed eyelids, which is generally thought to mean that something upsetting or incongruent is going on. As you see their eyes move you pace the behavior, "and perhaps during your experience today something I say causes some nervousness, or worry or something else ..." (I normally add a brief reframe then, for example, "and this usually means that your unconscious mind is very sensitive and discerning about new information, which is good ..."). When you pace any behavior in trance, reddening of your cheeks, a squirming in your chair, a smile, or a chuckle, some clients may get the idea that you can read their mind. If, in debriefing, you pick up on any negative feedback, verbal or non-verbal, explore it, process it, and put it to rest so it doesn't come back to plague you. If it's *not* there, no need to discuss it. Don't create a problem, just let the awe and mystery be your ally.

When doing hypnosis we often reach people very deeply. I estimate that rapport is accelerated ten times in hypnosis compared to conventional talk therapy. I am pleased and proud when someone is moved to say, "You touched my soul today," or even, "Wow, that was a cool experience!" Such intimacy was demonstrated to me one time when a woman, who had endured much misfortune and suffering in her life, was moved to tears of joy following a stock ego-strengthening story. I realized at that moment how this client had not only felt an embrace of her deepest self, but also how little positive regard she had experienced in her life.

This can be very gratifying for us as therapists. But the reaction of some clients can demonstrate the flip side, something I have witnessed a number of times. The client's reaction to hypnosis may have its positive aspects, they may be touched deeply, but when we try to process with them in the debriefing they are unable to articulate their thoughts and feelings. Their experience is novel – but also frightening, as it is beyond their reach, maybe something they believe they are not supposed to feel. We may then see a fear rush to the surface, as they are suddenly in unfamiliar territory. Explore it, process it, normalize it, and, if they want to continue, move on. My main point here is to anticipate the unexpected so it won't impede you doing your job.

Unconsciously directed hypnosis

We like to think that our everyday life is determined by deliberate choice or conscious intention; however, we are more often guided instead by features of the environment that operate outside of conscious awareness and control. Social psychologists have demonstrated that unconscious or automatic processes account for more of a person's mental functioning than was previously believed (Bargh and Chartrand, 1999). In other words, Milton Erickson had this right way back in 1930 when psychoanalysis ruled the day and when one's unconscious was regarded as a primordial ooze of negative impulses. Erickson recognized the unconscious as something positive and many writers since have employed the unconscious as a major target in therapy. The approach of this book is largely unconsciously directed; however, that doesn't mean that we should avoid *conscious* discussion and direction. To be sure, conscious discussion after trancework can help immensely in the integration of material. Also, many of the suggestions presented in the inductions in this book are indirect, as that is the way I generally work, and I provide a rationale for this.

However, there are plenty of times in therapy when I am highly directive, whether it's telling people to stop doing this or that, or "To get better you need to do X starting now," or even, "You don't need more therapy. You need to get a life!"

Hypnosis as adjunct

I have seen some clients for hypnosis where hypnosis was their only treatment, e.g., a person with no discernible disorder who wishes unconscious exploration for problem solving. However, I believe that in general if you are referred someone with an anxiety, mood, substance use, or other disorder, and the person eschews standard treatment, the magic bullet may be whizzing your way. Most clients I see are already in treatment elsewhere and they are referred for *adjunctive* treatment for anxiety or mood disorder, chronic pain, or insomnia. For example, the substance abuse treatment folks at Veterans Affairs had a young man whose substance abuse issues were stable, but he had nightmares that were immune to even strong medications like Seroquel. A few sessions of ego-strengthening plus the "amplifying the metaphor" technique cured the nightmares that were caused by childhood issues. Other people may be in individual or group therapy and many are on psychotropic medications. They are referred for hypnosis because the clients need something *in addition* to other treatment. The same is true for chronic pain clients who are typically involved in physical therapy, cognitive behavioral therapy (CBT), and medication. Following a few sessions of hypnosis, people often require less medication for pain. Clients referred for insomnia often cannot tolerate medications to aid sleep, or they request a "more natural" approach to combat insomnia.

What separates hypnosis – especially unconsciously directed hypnosis – from many other psychological treatments is that our target is the unconscious. I let them know right from the start that what may be holding them back is their unconscious mind, and that my therapeutic efforts will be directed at the big bull's eye which is "the back part of your mind." I also discuss with them realistic goals, e.g., a diminution of pain medication, or improving their sleep by an hour or two. To that end, whenever someone comes to me I'm thinking two major things, both of which we thank Milton Erickson for: (1) utilization, or *embracing* all that is involved in the client and his problem so I can *employ* these things in transforming the problem, and (2) pattern interruption, or interrupting some aspect of the problem, which can be the intensity, frequency, duration, location, or some other aspect (Cade and O'Hanlon, 1993). Of course, none of this is possible without a strong therapeutic relationship, and in this book I concentrate on what you can do to build your skills and confidence, which in turn will positively influence your client's trust and confidence in you.

What does the literature say about hypnosis?

The "ghost in the machine"

A burgeoning literature on neuroscience and hypnosis is now challenging the belief that the mind is merely "a ghost in the machine," as mental activities are bringing about physical changes that are far beyond the capabilities of a "ghost." In Los Angeles, Gary Wood and colleagues (2003) investigated the effect of hypnosis on psychoneuroimmunology. Study subjects received hypnotic induction, ego-strengthening suggestions, and suggestions for optimally balanced functioning of the immune and neuroendocrine systems. Blood samples drawn at five time points during the day yielded statistically significant immunological effects. Other studies using functional magnetic resonance imaging allow scientists to view brain activity that corresponds with hypnotic suggestion (Winerman, 2006), while other neuroimaging studies have used hypnotic suggestion to distinguish the brain structures most associated with sensory and affective dimensions of pain (Feldman, 2004).

Ernest Rossi (2003) extends Milton Erickson's "neuro-psycho-physiology" to current neuroscience research on activity dependent gene expression, neurogenesis, and stem cells in memory, learning, behavior change, and healing. He cites three conditions that can lead to the generation and maturation of new, functioning neurons in the adult brain: novelty, environmental enrichment, and exercise. Remember Samuel Johnson? His confidante and sidekick was Boswell. Well, Rossi was Erickson's Boswell (Jeff Zeig, personal communication, 1999). Rossi's books (Rossi, 2006; Rossi and Cheek, 1988) are rich reading, but even more of a treasure are his demonstrations at conferences, or video recordings of these experiences that are available from the Erickson Foundation. Indeed, the future of hypnosis is bright in terms of influencing the ghost's behavior as well as her molecules, cells, tissues, and organs (Dossey, 1999).

Gastrointestinal disorders

If I were to recommend an area of practice today, I would say, "Brush up on hypnosis and CBT and put yourself in a position to get referrals from a gastroenterologist practice in your area." Why? The strongest track record for hypnosis is with irritable bowel syndrome (IBS) (Whorwell, 2008). Gastrointestinal doctors know this and the general public is beginning to recognize it. Most gastrointestinal doctors would welcome someone like you who can help them with these problematic clients for whom medical treatment alone is of little help.

IBS is a functional gastrointestinal disorder characterized by abdominal pain, distention, and constipation, diarrhea, or both. It affects an estimated 10–20% of people worldwide (Tan, Hammond, and Gurala, 2005). The U.K. leads the way in demonstrating that hypnosis is a highly efficacious treatment, with improvement sustained for five years and longer (Whorwell, 2008). Were you to read only one paper on hypnosis and IBS, I recommend Gonsalkorale's (2006) paper that describes Whorwell's program at the University of Manchester.

In a world where CBT is a juggernaut, dominating the literature in the treatment of virtually all psychological disorders, the success of hypnosis with IBS is a rare exception. Of course, CBT remains a formidable treatment option (Blanchard, 2005). Recent researchers have demonstrated success combining CBT and hypnosis (Taylor, Read, and Hills, 2004; Golden, 2007). Hypnosis has shown promise in the treatment of other gastrointestinal disorders as well. Reflux esophagitis has responded well to hypnotic treatment (Zlotogorski and Anixter, 1983) as has functional dyspepsia (Kleibeuker and Thijs, 2004). In my current study (Fass, forthcoming) involving hypnosis and non-cardiac chest pain (NCCP) of esophageal origin, the treatment condition consists solely of ego-strengthening stories. The future may yield a further melding of CBT and hypnosis, as these potent modalities are applied in unison to the full range of functional gastrointestinal disorders.

Dermatology

Hypnosis also has a strong track record with certain derma-
tologic problems (Brown and Fromm, 1987; Spanos, Williams,
and Gwynn, 1990). Warts are especially susceptible to hypnosis (Lankton, 2007; Goldstein, 2005; Ewin, 1992). A psychologist friend, Bob Hall, and I saw a young Navajo Indian man
with HIV. His unsightly warts on hands and arms had been
unsuccessfully treated by cutting, burning, and freezing them
off. We offered him ego-strengthening stories and suggestions
for healing during three sessions over two months. After the
second session his skin began to clear. Following the third session he felt he was good to go, so we made him an audiotape for continued practice. Ten years later the warts were still
absent. In a follow-up phone call he said, "Whenever a wart
pops out, I pop in the tape." Philip Shenefelt (2004), a der-
matologist, has successfully used hypnosis with multiple skin
conditions including dermatitis, psoriasis, trichotillomania,
and post-herpetic neuralgia.

Other medical and surgical problems

Hammond (2008) reviewed the literature on the capability of
hypnosis to reduce inflammation, alter blood flow, and provide other beneficial effects. He provided historical examples
to show that hypnosis was the sole anesthetic for major surgeries dating to the 1800s. Recently at Walter Reed Army Medical
Center in the U.S. hypnosis was the sole anesthetic for septo-
plasty (Wain, 2004).

Olness (1980), in her study of pediatric cancer patients, cred-
ited hypnosis with a modification of the disease process itself.
Indeed, hypnosis with the terminally ill has been useful in
facilitating internal changes within certain patients who then
either recover completely, or who experience desirable life ex-
tension (Iglesias, 2004). In his case study of three end-stage,
terminally ill, adult cancer patients, Iglesias (2004) employed
hypnosis within existential psychotherapy. After six sessions
pain, nausea, and vomiting abated sufficiently to become re-
sponsive to medical management. Elkins et al. (2004) have

demonstrated the effectiveness of hypnosis in treating hot flashes in breast cancer survivors. Several years ago a psychotherapist at the M.D. Anderson Cancer Center in Houston told me of the staff's success with ego-strengthening stories in stabilizing mood and boosting hope. So, in many, many ways hypnosis can help improve quality of life – and then some – of cancer patients.

Ran Anbar, a pulmonologist and foremost U.S. expert on using hypnosis with pediatric pulmonary patients, has demonstrated the effectiveness of hypnosis with asthma, chest pain, cystic fibrosis, and other disorders (Anbar and Hummell, 2005). VandeVusse et al. (2007) showed that prenatal hypnosis preparation resulted in significantly less use of sedatives, analgesia, and regional anesthesia during labor and in higher one-minute Apgar scores. Daniel Araoz's groundbreaking book, *The New Hypnosis in Sex Therapy* (1998/1982) explicated the various applications of hypnosis in psychosexual disorders. In 2005 he expanded on this work by demonstrating the use of hypnosis in problems of gender identity, sexual orientation, and sexual preferences by using the client's imagery and inner resources to attain problem resolution (Araoz, 2005).

Various other conditions and disorders in dentistry, medicine, neurology, and surgery can be helped with hypnosis. But before we leave this section I wish to comment on how clients in trance may interpret what we say literally and concretely. Once I was seeing a man for headaches who had lost both legs to a land mine in World War II. Near the end of the session I offered him a restraining message, "a person shouldn't read too much into *hackneyed* metaphors." Suddenly he had phantom limb pain for the first time in years. He had no idea why, but I knew what it had to be. Fortunately it soon abated. Tailoring hypnosis to your client also encompasses what you *shouldn't* say, much like not emphasizing breathing when the person has lung disease.

:ing and weight management

ose of you in private practice, these referrals often comprise the majority of your clients. Working for the Veterans Affairs for many years I had the luxury of turning away those seeking the magic bullet. For weight loss referrals, I met with them and said, "I'll see you, but only after you meet with your dietitian and doctor and come back here with a plan for food and lifestyle change." Many never returned. Those who did come back knew that hypnosis was an adjunct and supportive of a larger program. Some lost weight and kept it off, others not. In a nutshell, if people are *ready* to change (Prochaska, DiClemente, and Norcross, 1992), whether it's tobacco cessation or weight management, hypnosis will likely help them, but so will nearly any other intervention. The person's stage of readiness is what's critical. Hypnosis can nudge clients toward desirable preparation and action stages (Gafner and Benson, 2003):

you know and I know that maintaining a healthy weight brings numerous health benefits, and I wonder what changes to your routine you might be contemplating now or in the near future ...

or:

seeing yourself in the future, you can notice how good it feels to be smoke-free, and when you can picture yourself as a non-smoker, in your mind, you will find yourself taking two nice, clean deep breaths ...

Clearly, there is a role for supportive hypnosis in habit control. Ego-strengthening, age regression, age progression, imaginal rehearsal, embedded suggestion, and other techniques can help motivate desired change and sustain it once it has been achieved. I saw smokers only after they had completed a stop smoking class. I realize that folks in private practice may approach it differently, and I respect that. For you, I believe that your success will be greater if hypnosis is an adjunct. Kirsch, Montgomery, and Sapirstein (1995) underscored that the *addi-*

tion of hypnosis to CBT leads to sustained weight loss when compared to CBT alone. *The Thin Book* (Brickman, 2000) is an excellent resource for weight management; however, I have also used its tenets and phrasing for other problems.

"No brain, no pain": issues of chronic pain

Milton Erickson was said to have noted something like, "Place one foot in the patient's world, but always keep one foot planted in your own world." I remember the *Star of India* docked in San Diego. It was secured with a really thick rope. I imagine that rope around one of my ankles when working with chronic pain clients. If only we could simply apply our myriad hypnotic techniques like transforming the symptom ("your searing discomfort can begin to feel like the drumming of warm little fingers on your lower back ...") and people could cope better with their awful pain. However, the situation is often complicated by guilt, blame, secondary gain, relational issues, opioid dependence, a cornucopia of comorbid psychological disorders, the compounding problems of old age, and other factors. So, then, can hypnosis help these clients? You bet! It may be hard to believe, but these are actually my favorite clients because of their complexity and because so many hypnotic techniques can be successfully applied to them. Ego-strengthening as a foundation, unconscious exploration and problem solving where indicated, utilization, the liberal application of hypnotic language and embedded suggestion, and a variety of pain-specific techniques are a few of the things we can employ with these clients. Adjunctive hypnosis is especially applicable here, as clients hopefully also will be participating in a CBT or support group in addition to medical therapies.

Some in the U.S. view chronic pain as woefully *under*-treated, whether with medications or techniques like hypnosis (Patterson et al., 2004). So, when I'm treating a client who does not have secondary gain or personality disorder and who either does not respond to treatment, or who triggers in me the thought that something else is going on here, I first suspect either under-treated depression or pain. An excellent paper on treating chronic pain is Mark Jensen's "The neurophysiology of pain perception and hypnotic analgesia: Implications for clinical practice" (2008). A few of the take-home messages for the practitioner include: (1) The "side effects" of hypnotic analgesia are overwhelmingly positive even though we don't yet know which hypnotic interventions or suggestions are most effective, or which suggestions are more effective for which conditions. (2) Useful are suggestions for dissociation and a "special place," age regression and age progression, acceptance strategies, and cognitive restructuring. (3) Suggestions should address pain intensity, location, and quality, as well as pleasurable and calm physical sensations.

Another must-have paper for someone who treats pain is Jeffrey Feldman's "Expanding hypnotic pain management to the affective dimension of pain" (2009). As with the Jensen article, I'll omit the neuroscience due to space limitations and offer a few of his key points for the clinician: (1) Frame hypnosis as impacting both sensation and affect. (2) Inquire about the current level of both sensation and affect. (3) Utilize inductions, suggestions, and posthypnotic suggestions that address both. (4) Emphasize wording that targets the most relevant emotion – anger, sadness, or anxiety. Gafner and Benson's *Hypnotic Techniques* (2003) has a large chapter on treating pain, as well as the resources listed at the end of this book.

Insomnia

Like chronic pain and some psychological disorders, insomnia referrals may result when other practitioners become frustrated or aggravated with these clients' lack of progress. Some with insomnia may have un/under-treated depression or chronic pain. Whether they have difficulty getting to sleep, staying asleep, or waking up too early in the morning, one of these clients' chief problems is rumination. They don't drink coffee after noon, the bedroom is quiet, ear plugs keep out the barking dogs, progressive muscle relaxation has relaxed the body, but that darn busy mind just won't shut off. What a great target here, the unconscious mind! As with pain, pattern interruption applies, as well as having a realistic goal of diminution of the symptom rather than the total elimination of it.

I have treated many insomnia cases, usually with three to four sessions. I make them a tailored CD to listen to before bed, and I estimate that 60% received some benefit. I have a discussion on the disorder along with various sleep inductions in *More Hypnotic Inductions* (Gafner, 2006).

Substance abuse

At one time in the U.S. hypnotic treatment of alcoholism was quite popular. In the 1800s success rates as high as 80% with samples of up to 700 were reported (Martensen, 1997). By 1920, though, hypnosis had developed an unsavory reputation due to its use in entertainment. Fast forward to 2009 and we see that hypnosis is now making a comeback in the addiction field. Walsh (2003) reported success with cocaine addicts with his Utilization Sobriety model that employs ideomotor finger signals. In his study that involved highly intensive (20 daily sessions) of hypnotic treatment with adult clients who were primarily alcohol dependent, Potter (2004) reported a success rate of 77% after one year.

Ronald Pekala, a noted researcher and psychologist at the Veterans Affairs in Coatesville, Pennsylvania, is a longtime proponent of ego-strengthening in hypnosis and psychotherapy. His study (Pekala et al., 2004) involving 261 veterans with drug and alcohol dependence found that subjects who listened to a self-hypnosis audiotape improved significantly in self-esteem and anger/impulsivity compared to the other two treatment conditions. Clearly, in the burgeoning field of addictions, traditional treatment modalities are making room for hypnosis as an efficacious treatment. In the coming years hypnosis practitioners should have a cornucopia of opportunity in this field.

Anxiety and mood disorders

In treating post-traumatic stress disorder (PTSD), I have used hypnosis primarily with combat veterans, women and men who were sexually assaulted in the military, and torture survivors at a refugee clinic (Gafner and Benson, 2001).

23

Hypnosis is very helpful in containing toxic emotion, diminishing insomnia, reframing traumatic memories, and overall stress management. Due to demand for PTSD treatment in the Veterans Affairs oftentimes clients must wait to begin comprehensive treatment. Accordingly, hypnotic treatment can help clients manage symptoms while they are waiting. Sperr and Hyer (1994) noted that in their work with combat veterans, the main value of hypnosis is its ability to aid the client in finding a better perspective on some dimension of the trauma experience. Kingsbury (1988) stated that the pathological symptoms of PTSD, such as dissociation and numbing, are also common phenomena in hypnosis. Because of this natural "fit," he called hypnosis an isomorphic intervention for PTSD. Schoenberger (2000) did a meta-analysis of CBT treatments for anxiety disorders. In many of the studies, subjects who received hypnosis in addition to CBT showed significant improvement compared to those who received CBT alone. So, again, the take-home message here is hypnosis as adjunct.

Hypnosis can be of major assistance with the self-regulation of panic disorder (Iglesias and Iglesias, 2005). This report, like the majority touting the value of hypnosis with generalized anxiety disorder (GAD) and other anxiety disorders, consist mainly of case reports. Some dismiss case reports; however, in them we may discover novel techniques and approaches to clinical problems. One major value is their inclusion of hypnosis *combined with* other techniques, for example, hypnosis and rational emotive behavior therapy, or hypnosis and acupuncture. Gordon and Gruzelier (2003) describe their work with a ballet dancer in which they combine hypnosis and neurolinguistic programming, and Poon (2009) relates in her case study her phase-oriented treatment with four traumatized Chinese women. Indeed, this is rich clinical material not likely to be found in a randomized clinical trial!

In our hypnosis training group in Tucson we fielded many referrals for anxiety disorders. This included GAD, social phobia, panic disorder, and adjustment disorder. Many referrals came from the psychotic disorders program where the most common Axis I disorder was paranoid schizophrenia. These clients' psychotic disorder was stable; however, they required assistance with secondary anxiety. We found story techniques especially helpful. This included a "straight forward" story with its attendant meta-messages, as well as story within a story, alternating stories, and story without an ending. We would tailor therapy to the person, determine which techniques generated the most positive response, see them for three to six sessions, make them an individualized tape or CD, and then send them on their way. As with many other disorders, building a foundation with ego-strengthening was inestimably valuable, as oftentimes clients may not be willing to give up their symptoms until they feel strong enough to do so.

Yexley (2007) demonstrated the efficacy of hypnosis in treating postpartum depression. Yapko (1992, 2001), on whom Yexley leans heavily in planning treatment, is the foremost advocate of employing hypnotic strategies in the treatment of depression and related mood disorders. He draws upon social psychology, CBT, hypnosis, and other areas for background and development of treatment. He zeroes in on *frame of reference* and *choice* as he builds a momentum of responsiveness. Indeed, with depression even more than with other disorders, hypnotic phenomena can be utilized and reframed. To cite but one example, rigidity, which is actually catalepsy, that inexorable suspension of movement – psychologically, behaviorally, physiologically, and socially – can be countered by suggestions of fluidity and flexibility. Yapko's books and CDs are superb examples of employing the best of CBT, hypnosis, metaphor, and strategic psychotherapy.

Yapko and others are influenced by the work of Milton Erickson, whose approach is seen in one of his signature techniques, the rehearsal technique in working with dreams hypnotically (Edgette and Edgette, 1995). With it, the client verbally processes the dream (or fantasy) with a different cast of characters, different setting, different outcome, and so on, but with the same meaning. This is repeated again and again as needed. And you thought that this technique was thought up by the originators of trauma incident reduction!

Looking beyond mere technique, we see that this approach to hypnotic dreaming embodies Erickson's belief that a major way we can help people is by making something that is static into something fluid and dynamic, thus effecting a critical reframe and transforming the problem. To Erickson, the meaning of the dream and the person's understanding of it was secondary to turning a frozen experience into something that could flow and evolve. We should keep this in mind as a general principle as we apply hypnotic techniques to the myriad problems we see in our practices. In their excellent paper, Lynn and Hallquist (2004) dissect Erickson's strategies and tactics, which they explain primarily in terms of response set theory.

To measure or not

I frequently use pre- and post-measures for depression, anxiety, and self-efficacy. I will also get a 0–10 report from the client to gauge progress. I believe that if we never use any paper-and-pencil measures we are open to valid criticism. Someone once said that scientists measure and everything else is just poetry. Some rely heavily on hypnotic susceptibility scales and make a good case for doing so, while many others, including myself, do not.

The hypnosis setting

You want hypnosis to be something that is warm, inviting, and welcoming. To that end, your office should be a sanctuary, a comfortable place that is different from the sterile office or group room that clients often come to expect in a clinical setting. To me, low light is essential, so I usually have one or two lamps that I can turn on when any overhead lights are turned off. Pictures or posters on the walls are a nice touch, as well as a rug on the floor. A recliner allows people to put up their feet. Some people may prefer to sit in a straight-backed chair or love seat. In times when I've had an office on a busy corridor I've placed a Sound Screen outside the door. I usually play a CD of relaxing music, wind chimes music, or something similar. I especially like Liquid Mind, an excellent background sound.

During the first session I usually ask clients what I can do to help them feel comfortable, and to do whatever they need to do for their maximum comfort. Accordingly, the setting, like therapy, is geared to the individual. Be prepared for some people to take you at your word when you give them license to be comfortable. One man sauntered over to my desk, sat in the chair, propped his feet on the desk and said, "Okay, let's get started." That was the only time I saw that guy. No shortage of Axis II in the Veterans Affairs. One man, who weighed 300 pounds, cleared a place in the room and lay down on the floor. He readily went into a very nice trance; however, I had to enlist the help of two others to get him up afterward. In the following sessions he sat in a chair like everyone else.

Remember to turn off all pagers and phones, put a Do Not Disturb sign on your door, and you're ready to create a most memorable experience for you and your client.

3. Story Inductions

Story Inductions

Glen Canyon

In a moment I will read you an account of floating down the Colorado River in 1963 before the gates of Glen Canyon dam closed and water from the river began to fill in this 200-mile expanse. I call this account My Journey of Discovery and some listeners of this story have indeed discovered something of importance in their own lives. You may sit back, close your eyes if you wish, and let yourself travel in your own way as I read you the following induction.

I want to tell you about time, both clock time and geologic time, *rapidly occurring* time distortion *time* like the shutter speed of my camera, and *timeless time*, like when the photo of shimmering sandstone cliffs remains in my mind's eye. Or, when the camera's tripod waits on the soft sand of the river's shore, *time standing still*, awaiting ephemeral light and shadow for the next photograph, milliseconds blending into minutes amidst millennia's majesty. How delightful when my *unmoving body* and *steady gaze* are *arrested* by vermillion cliffs, or when an *hour escapes* my grasp, and the sun descends in mere *seconds*, when mid-afternoon *hurtles* into nighttime as my eyes briefly close. I remember well *the grave of the Confederate soldier* near Pick Axe Canyon, and how each year I would pause there and *see new pieces* of gray uniform that were brought up by pack rats. Wherever we stop for the night along the river the stars are so bright I can read by them, but after a few words *sleep* comes quickly and the images of the day are woven into my *dreams*.

Dreaming by night and journeying as if in a dream by day, therein my travels through Glen Canyon. One minute my body is *heavy*, warmed by the sun, though my mind is *light*, and the next minute alternating air currents – *moist, dry, cool, warm* – enliven my body as my mind is seized by the vibrant *green* of a *red*bud tree, and behind that green the delicate lavender of the walls gives way to slate gray and powder blue sky, and then to black because a crow has cawed somewhere. I can hear my breathing in that narrow canyon, and my footfalls produce an echo on the crackling shale, but soon my feet, *way down there*, are back on soft river sand.

It is time to leave this lovely canyon, knowing I will return, if only in my dream. My body moves on, *disconnected* from my mind way back there, as the ever-beckoning river awaits and my journey continues. I most

Marginal annotations:
- time distortion
- catalepsy eye fixation
- time distortion
- fluff
- suggestions
- apposition of opposites
- dissociation
- dissociation

appreciate this trip late in the year when long shadows and subdued light make the best photos. Late in the year the sun drops quickly behind the walls and the *chill* of apposition of opposites my body is embraced by the *warmth* of the campfire. Driftwood burns hot and fast, as do rock – hard chunks of juniper – spiraled, twisted, ancient. *Sleep* descends rapidly, suggestion as we are lulled by the waves lapping the shore, the crackling fire, and then comes the stillness.

We embark at Mexican Hat and we float between gray limestone walls and towering cliffs of Navajo sandstone. At Rosebud Canyon a spring high above cascades down, giving life to a hanging garden of trees, flowers, mosses, and ferns. It is a good place to stop for the night. We leave the raft, stretch, and briefly explore petroglyphs left by the ancients. We see something we have found in many canyons, Kokopelli, the hunchback flute player. *Sleep* arrives even suggestions earlier this evening, and soon we *drift and dream*. I awake in the middle of the night – what time could it be? I do not know, as no one wears a watch – and I *walk woodenly* catalepsy into a canyon. I hear a chorus of frogs that I did not notice before. The moonlight casts a blue scrim over the petroglyphs, and the jagged cliffs now appear soft and as if in motion. *Is that* a human figure up ahead? positive hallucinations I look back to where I remember the river to be, and I see a sheet of molten silver. Did *someone* call my name? *I hear* a lilting flute above the canyon. Many feelings and images reverberate within me now as I write this account, memories resurfacing from an unknown stimulus. Now at home the morning sun's kiss is *warm* on my face as I apposition of opposites gaze out the kitchen window, and the *cold* tap water brings back *burning* sun on my bare shoulder as we wade through trenches of *chilly* water near Rainbow Bridge, my body as heavy as the boulders around me. The *coldness* disappears as I glimpse the ancient sand dunes up ahead, inviting, *warm*, embracing.

Mystery Canyon was so named because steps carved into the wall end half-way up, and no one knows what can be found way up at the top. The falling water echoes softly in the pools at the bottom where we lay by the campfire, and we are playing a guessing game. "It is the remnant of a lost civilization, the Mystery People of Mystery Canyon," someone ventures. "When I close my eyes I can hear their words, way up there," says another. "It's the Sand Man, that's who's up there," I whisper, and soon we are fast *asleep*.   suggestion

Twilight Canyon leads to a large amphitheater that could accommodate a thousand people. All around the bottom are pictographs: mountain goats, the sun, and stick figure people whose *feet are absent*. "Where   dissociation did the feet go?" someone asks. "*Disconnected, off somewhere*," I answer. Another responds, "It reminds me of the unseen hand, or maybe one hand not clapping," as we move deeper into the vast amphitheater, an awesome and incredible place. At the exit near the back we pass through a narrow aperture and gaze up at a beautiful smooth wall with a natural design in the rock. With a little imagination *we see* a chariot pulled   positive hallucinations by horses, their manes flying in the breeze.

Sometime later we find ourselves at Music Temple. "J. W. Powell, 1869," is among the names we find inscribed on the wall. I re- member reading the 1871 account of John Wesley Powell, who *lost an arm* in the Civil   dissociation War. He wrote about the "sweet sounds" of Music Temple, a vast hollow space where this night we light a candle. We close our eyes and *hear* in 1957 the water dripping – I know not from where – and *imagine* in   positive hallucination this great cathedral the same symphony heard by Powell nearly a century ago. Be- fore the candle burns down I take my party to a recess in the wall. I reach in and ex- tract a pot. I hold it in my hands and say, "Notice the distinctive whorl of the corn flower. Anthropologists say this was made by someone they call Corn Woman in the late Anasazi period. Her design has been found on similar pots from Chaco Canyon to northern Mexico." The others caress the pot before I return it to its ledge. The can- dle is now extinguished and our feet barely touch the ground as we glide out of Music Temple, *forgetting* if day or night awaits us   amnesia on the exterior.

That night by the campfire someone says, "I now know what it means when 'scien- tists can see through time.'" Late that night I steal from my sleeping bag. In the lemon glow beside the river a stick finds its way to my hand. The stick moves *of its own accord*   automatic drawing in the sand. Whether my hand drew a corn flower or something else, or if this in fact occurred in my dream, I do not know.
Source: Nichols (2000).

Deepening

Beginning now, I would like you to allow your experience to deepen as I count backward from 10 down to 1, starting to count now 10, ... 9, ... 8, ...

Notes for practice

After realerting your client it is important for you to ask some specific questions while they are still feeling the effects of trance. I customarily ask, "How much time do you think passed since you came in here?" Many will guess either more or less time has elapsed, and I then say, "Good, that's time distortion." I also ask, "How do you feel in your hands and feet?" People typically respond with tingling or numbness, coldness or warmth, or lightness or heaviness. Such hypnotic phenomena need to be elicited so they can be ratified. Some clients' response is light or subtle and these folks need reinforcement in order to understand that they experienced trance. When I notice facial mask, lack of swallowing, or body immobility, I comment on it. This education process is vital, especially in the first session. If you don't ask the right questions and point out where time distortion, dissociation, and other phenomena occurred, they might say, "I don't think I went under." The corollary of not feeling anything is, "I didn't experience hypnosis, so why should I return?" For sure, a minority of clients' response is light. For them, reinforce what they *did* experience.

You learn many important things during debriefing of the first session. Could they hear you okay? Hearing loss occurs even in young people. Some hearing loss, not apparent during conversation when they can see your face, may show itself as you speak softly during hypnosis when their eyes are closed. You may need to use an audio amplifier next time. "Oh, I hated that background music," they might say, or, "You mentioned a lake, I almost drowned in a lake one time." All this is vital data on which you build in subsequent sessions.

Contest of Time

As I read you the following induction about time – and losing track of time – you may settle into that chair, close your eyes if you wish, and pay attention to this curious story about time. It was October 2005 and *outside* it was brisk. The fallen leaves crunched crisply beneath one's feet, but *inside* the old metropolitan edifice several hundred patrons of the arts in period costumes were gathered for what had become known as the Annual Contest of Time. Three people dressed in early 1600's garb sat on stage. Their names had been drawn from several hundred who had submitted their names for the contest. The audience eagerly awaited the start of this year's prestigious plenary contest.

The contestants' names had been drawn from a 1603 copper vat reputed to have been owned by Oliver Cromwell. Phoebe Ingersoll, president of the Greater Philadelphia Time Piece Society, announced, "In Cromwell's vat we have placed precisely 375 names, and at the conclusion of tonight's event we will know which one of our three contestants is this year's winner." The audience gazed down at the stage which had been assembled in the former medical school amphitheater. Phoebe paused a moment before continuing. "In years past momentous surgeries were performed in this very place, and this evening's operation will be no less compelling. These three contestants, as you can see, are seated amidst five of the most valuable antiquarian clocks in existence. The winner of our contest becomes the owner of these clocks, collectively appraised last year at over half a million U.S. dollars."

The lights dimmed. Large portraits of Benjamin Rush, Galen, and Maimonedes were now barely discernible on the walls. A digital clock on stage was set at zero minutes zero seconds.

Phoebe continued, "The rules of the contest are thus. Our participants, who will soon have their eyes covered, will listen closely as our moderator offers a brief history of these time pieces. As you know, this will be a pure test of *time distortion*, that intriguing phenomenon whereby a person *loses track of time*. The contestant who comes closest to guessing the elapsed time will be our winner. Ladies and gentlemen, affix your eye covers *now*. Time keeper, please start the clock. Let's welcome our horological interpreter, Sir Winston Ingot." A polite applause followed.

Ingot began his patter in a rich, melodious voice that enveloped his listeners, immediately arresting their attention. "I am privileged to stand beside the so-called Cromwell Family Clock, built by John Fromantel in London in 1673. Its height is 79 inches with a depth of 15 and 3/4 inches. Kind audience, if only you could reach down from up there and caress this beautiful burl walnut veneer on oak, its gilt and silvered metal and glass. I will pause for *nine seconds* so that you might hear its determined tick …, oh, 6.5 seconds will have to suffice. Lore of the day had Cromwell lifting its hood to wind it one evening. He reached inside and abruptly paused, his mind having evidently drifted to some faraway place. Cromwell remained in this dream world for several minutes, we are told. When awakened by his wife he reported, 'My mind is a feather, my body of lead, a most wonderful reverie.' The fact that Cromwell evidently expired *before* the clock was built only serves to deepen both the mystery and our reverence for this clock, which continues to absorb our curiosity, as well as our fascination with *elusive time*, after more than three *centuries* – and not to mention nearly incalculable *seconds and minutes*."

Sir Winston inhaled deeply before continuing. "Kind audience, I draw much inspiration from these astounding time pieces and I invite you now to enjoy some cool, refreshing breaths as we resume our journey from the 1600s to the present and back again, when in real time and space these four clocks are placed but a few feet from each other and as far as several meters from the back row of this wonderful amphitheater." He gazed down at his feet for what *seemed like* two or three minutes but which, in reality, was but several long seconds. He began to speak again with his head still inclined. "Kind audience, very often during these contests people doze off during my boring monologue. Believe me, it took years of practice to become this *boring*. In fact, I fell asleep once myself, right here one time, and I was swaying on my feet until someone from the back row yelled, 'Time is of the essence, Ingot!' That was followed by the muttering of an impatient woman who said, 'Save the golden gift of sleep for later, Sir Winston,' and I woke up *sooner* than an Oklahoma Sooner, quickly realizing that this was Pennsylvania in the 21st century." Then he paused again, this time for what was actually *five minutes* or more.

"Our curiosity in such time pieces continues centuries later – let me count, 1673, 1773, 1873, 1973, all the way up to the present year of 2005, exactly how many years is that?" he whispered. The audience showed rapt attention for his words, as people inclined themselves forward. One woman, who sat cross-legged in the aisle, muttered to no one in particular, "It has taken no time at all for both my legs to fall completely *asleep*." Sir Winston continued, "From the 1600s to the present and back again, something you may feel in your mind or your body, these four beautiful clocks, separated from each other by mere inches but joined by the wonderful art of clock making across several *centuries of time* ..." and his voice drifted off again. He spoke louder when he resumed. "In the audience you can caress with your eyes these remarkable time pieces, while our contestants, with their eyes essentially closed, must employ their imaginations to discern the details. One contestant one time remarked, 'I go *deep inside* when my eyes are closed. I first regarded the experience as interesting, then curious, and eventually realized that this internal focus was splendidly *intriguing*.'

Ingot then gestured to someone off to the side, and immediately the lights dimmed further. The timepieces were at once bathed in a lavender light, and flute and wind chime music emanated from speakers somewhere, precisely where it was difficult to determine. A woman contestant adjusted herself in her chair, her head inclined forward, and soon she was fast asleep. Ingot inhaled deeply and once again his deep voice resounded. This moment would later be described by Phoebe Ingersoll as "a most precious and memorable *gateway moment* when *time* on earth was *frozen*, and when an angel seemed to pass over."

Another pause from Ingot was followed by, "We now turn our attention to our first time piece known as A Clock for the Rooms by John Child of Philadelphia. Notice the exquisite Roman numerals and the highly polished maple cabinet. Notes from the Logan Library indicate that a fire in 1796 or 1797 destroyed many clocks save this one which was scarred by flames. A most bizarre phenomenon is this: where the flames seared the cabinet it remains – to this day – warm to the touch." He gently took the hand of the contestant nearest the clock and placed her hand on the cabinet's side and commanded, "Feel the centuries' warmth, madam." The woman quickly pulled her hand away but the hand remained in the air, floating with a seeming life of its own. "A veritable autonomy in that warm hand, madam," he whispered. This contestant, too, was soon asleep, but her hand remained extended in the air.

"Audience, you are so kind to endure my palling patter, and I don't mind one bit if you, too, doze off. In fact, I too fell asleep one time after caressing the warmth of the Child Clock, as it beckoned a pleasant experience from my own childhood. The third and fourth clocks I shall survey in a more cursory manner, as more time has passed than we had planned on." His pause was briefer this time. "Regard the famous William Penn Clock," he said. "It is by William Martin of Bristol from 1700. In this English tall case pendulum clock the pendulum is said to weigh 15 pounds, but when held in the hand 'feels light as nearly a bundle of feathers,' according to archives at Pennsbury Manor. One winding permits flawless time keeping for a full thirty days. You may note that absent from tonight's discussion is *escapement*, an essential feature in many clocks. I know that a *mental escape* can be a highly pleasant *temporal experience*, but we do indeed need to concentrate on elapsed time in this contest."

Sir Winston continued, "The next clock was donated to the Logan Library in 1904 by descendants of Edward Duffield, who was known as Benjamin Franklin's clockmaker. Duffield was a close personal friend of Franklin for thirty years, according to one source, thirty-seven years according to another. This eight-foot tall walnut Queen Anne clock case houses a brass arched dial. It is designed to ring at *sunup* and *sundown* and its chapter ring center is matted in a concentric pattern." Sir Winston gestured again. The music stopped, the lavender light dissipated, and the auditorium was returned to bright light. "What about the other clock?" someone asked. "Unfortunately we *don't have time* for it," answered Ingot. Phoebe Ingersoll grasped a dark cloth and covered the digital clock that had been running since the start of the contest. Each contestant was handed a 5 x 7 inch card and a magic marker. Ingot's voice boomed, "Contestants, before your eye coverings are removed I want you to record your *estimate of elapsed time*." Two contestants awoke with a start. "Quick, now, write the *time*," instructed Sir Winston.

The drape covering the digital clock was yanked away. The time read 58 minutes, 20 seconds. One contestant's card revealed *34 minutes, zero seconds*, the closest to the elapsed time. As Phoebe Ingersoll was about to announce the winner, the William Penn clock chimed *one time*, a reverberating ring that transported all from the *here-and-now*.
Source: Stiefel (2006).

Deepening

Beginning now, I would like you to picture in your mind a large, old fashioned clock with three hands. You can see in your mind, the second hand moving, a bit at a time, and as you do so, you can let your experience deepen. After a minute or so I will resume speaking again.

Notes for practice

In the induction some references to time, as well as time distortion, are underscored along with a few key suggestions. Let's say this is an initial hypnosis session with a client. You will want to ask her about any time distortion, but also about other hypnotic phenomena. Interestingly, I have found that some clients' response to this induction involves other phenomena, but no time distortion at all! Did you employ a slight vocal alteration for key suggestions? How about your rate while reading? In my experience many people new to hypnosis will read way too fast. Alter your rate, maybe slower one paragraph, then a bit faster the next. Indeed, clients will tell you things like, "You spoke too fast." We glean many important things during the debriefing. Did you look up from the script sufficiently to monitor the client's ongoing response? If the person had shifted in her chair at some point, could you have deviated from the script in order to pace the behavior, e.g., "and certainly today you can do anything necessary to feel more comfortable ..." To be sure, many times such a comment may not be necessary.

Critique the way you conducted the session. If your therapy component consisted of a long story, did you leave enough time for debriefing? Is this an induction that can become a stock induction for your repertoire, one that you can ad lib one day without reading? With practice your comfort will grow and this will translate as confidence to your client.

Redwall

As I read you the following I'd like you to sit back, close your eyes if you wish, and begin to contemplate openness, yes, openness to new experience. Who knows what a person can experience on an unconscious level?

The Redwall is like a Great Wall of China, thousands of miles of palisade that wraps in and out of the Grand Canyon in Arizona. It allows few ways up or down, past or through, and any exit may mean descending to the Colorado River far below. Any ascending or descending routes are where the rock has broken apart, difficult to find faults or fractures.

I am here at Redwall and I cannot find my way through. No guidebook explains the way. I am in a limestone-walled side canyon below the south rim of the Canyon. This rock walkway hangs like a high wire, a thin passageway carved into rock between pearl-smooth walls. I peer down a 700-foot drop. This natural barrier of cliffs between the upper and lower regions of the Grand Canyon has stymied me again. Whatever will I do? After two days I finally succeed in finding an exit, and right then I promise myself I will be better prepared before I venture in here another time.

That is why, on a blazing hot June day in 1999, I find myself in Phoenix, Arizona, to see a legendary outdoorsman. I have read everything I could put my hands on about Redwall, inquired among tour guides and hikers, and one name has come up time and time again: Sigfried Gunter. This man is known for discovering 116 different passages during 12,000 miles of hiking the Canyon over forty-two years.

His home is a modest duplex in south Phoenix. As I near the door I discern something scrawled into the cement next to the welcome mat. It is the word "discover." I ring the doorbell and wait for what seems like the longest time. As I peer through the screen door into a dark room I hear, "Young lady, I wonder if you realize that right now you are close to South Mountain." "I didn't know that," I answer to the voice in the dark. The man's voice then adds, "It all depends on where you are looking from. The Indians south of here call it North Mountain." I answer, "Yes, perspective is what you mean." "Looking toward, seeking, and discovery may not have much in common," says the voice. This time I don't know how to answer.

The voice speaks again. "Enter at your own risk, young woman. I can tell you must be searching for something." A small, wiry man in his nineties suddenly materializes from the dark. The door swings open before I can introduce myself. Determined eyes meet mine as he extends a gnarled and calloused hand. I follow him as he says over his shoulder, "Just call me Gunter. Let's sit in the backyard, it's cooler there." He leads me through the dark living room filled with bird cages. The birds chortle and ruffle their feathers. Behind me a large dog barks. In the kitchen I hear the scurrying of small animals over tile. "It's also quieter out in back," he says. Gunter gestures me to a lawn chair. Three ceiling fans whir above me. I smell green chilies grilling nearby. Is that Mexican Norteno music emanating from the adjoining yard? Piles of books lay about the screened-in porch. "Each one of those books is on either mathematics or chess," he ventures absentmindedly. "Many have asked me if I use mathematics or chess to find my way in the Canyon and the answer is maybe," he remarks.

He takes a seat slightly behind and to the left of me. "I have very old eyes, lady," he says. His voice is like sandpaper on stucco. He adds, "Side vision only, and all this you may soon disregard, simply forget, or just not see, time will tell." I am perplexed by these words and am not sure how to respond. "When you called you said your name was Beth, is that right?" Before I can answer he says, "You're pretty brave just walking in here to see a strange old man. Care for a nice, cold lemonade?" He has already disappeared into the darkness of the kitchen. Two years later I would experience a burst of creativity and a sense of discovery whenever I sipped a lemonade.

But for now, seated in the comfort of the screen porch, my mind dreams, and in my mind I have suddenly drifted to the Canyon. My body has assumed a most incredible levity, and heat and abundance surge from deep within. One second I am floating above the Colorado River and a millisecond later I find myself down below, immersed in the geometry and kaleidoscope of colors amidst the rocks. I am at once up there and down here, and it is a most enjoyable juxtaposition of sensations. In my misty reverie I hear incandescent words that paraphrase the words of another, "I am light therefore I am ever so lost in levity." A powerful acceptance embraces me, acceptance of precisely what I do not know, nor does it matter.

A billowy breeze buffets my hair as if I am in a wind tunnel. My finger traces a deer on the sandstone, a pictograph of the ancients. A cactus wren chirps loudly from somewhere and then I am soaring again. Are those eagles or hawks down below? The river is a chromatic brown thread and I can see for miles and miles.

I am down below now amidst the rocks. It is a dreamy slot canyon. My heart beats wildly as I am clutched in the preciousness of life. I reach out. The stone feels rough – sandstone, limestone, it does not matter – and my hand reaches out. Fingers extend and crinkle the leaves of a bush. The sweet scent of the leaves is soon doused by splashing river water. I caress the colossal rock formation, sand grain details, and each crevice takes on meaning. Every rock is rich in implication and I ponder scouring floods of eons past. My hand grasps a dry gourd and I shake it hard. Is there a rhythm in the seeds? Where do I go next – do I stay right here or do I float again above the clouds? Destination is of no import as my absorption deepens in time future, time present, and past, and a cascade of sensations embraces me.

Once again I sense that body of mine in its lawn chair. My nose detects green peppers grilling, tumbling, churning, and an accordion in the music beckons, pulsating on the right side, while the left side of me senses birds chortling, more scurrying of busy animal feet across tile, and then cold water – not cold like river water – but something cold and glassy, frosty in my palm, and my opening eyes take in a lemonade being nudged into my hand. "I hope you like it with lots of ice and not too sweet," intones a voice.

We sit for maybe thirty minutes, each sipping our lemonades. Finally I ask, "What was the subject of your doctoral dissertation?" "Spiral helices in Euclidian space," he answers. I say, "I thought you said mathematics didn't help you with Redwall." "I didn't say that exactly, did I?"

I feel it is time to press on. "You've heard of the fabled Via Regia, the Royal Road through Redwall?" I ask. "Yup." "You've probably been there, too, am I right?" I ask. "Maybe." People had told me visiting him might be frustrating. Long, awkward seconds tick by.

Finally he says, "Beth, whenever I'm at Redwall I ponder only two things: pattern and design, and I ask myself, 'What is the order in this chaos?' And then I find my way. Ready for another lemonade?"

Once again he has disappeared before I can answer. I sit back in the lawn chair, somehow sinking deeper this time, and I drift and dream.
Source: Childs (2001).

Deepening

As your experience deepens, I would like your unconscious mind to once again contemplate the idea of openness, yes, receptivity to openness and novel experience. All this may occur as I tell you a little story about Sandra, who one evening solved a puzzle during her dream.

Sandra had a rather hectic and pressure-filled work and personal life and she had welcomed her vacation at the Wunderbar Castle in Germany. After a long day of sightseeing she lay down in front of the fireplace and soon was fast asleep. In her dream she saw herself hard at work trying to solve a particular task, which was, in this castle, how to go from room to room.

Her mind reviewed the numerous ways she could get from here to there. She could simply walk from one room to another. She could go outside, cross the moat, return and then go from one room to another. She could walk in briskly, amble in slowly; enter the room in the morning, afternoon, or the evening. She could go in on the half hour, on the quarter hour, crawl in on her belly, shimmy in on her back; go in with one station playing on the radio, or have her favorite CD playing while she went in. She could enter after drinking coffee or tea with sugar or milk, or after drinking Diet Pepsi, or any other number of beverages. She could go outside and ride a horse and then enter the room, or take a taxi cab to Berlin, fly to Bismarck, North Dakota and back and then go from one room to another. She could put on shorts or a dress, wait until the evening, go outside and enter through the window, and then go from one room to another.

As her dream deepened she continued to review all the possible ways to get from here to there, and finally, after seemingly endless unconscious deliberation, she realized that there were really innumerable ways to go from one room to another.

Notes for practice

Many of our clients are stuck and keep doing the same thing over and over again. To me, this is a therapeutic invitation to perturb; in other words, to help them break up unwelcome and all too familiar dysfunctional patterns. A major way I perturb is through instigative stories and anecdotes (Gafner, 2004). The story above, Wunderbar Castle, is adapted from two other stories, Going from Room to Room, a Milton Erickson teaching tale in Rosen (1982), and Simple Rooms (Gafner, 2004).

Clients could be stuck in depression, an unsatisfying job, or unsatisfactory relationship. Or they could be existentially bogged down in general. Now, a cognitive behavioral therapist who sees such clients may spend a session or two clarifying the goal before beginning active intervention. A psychiatrist may value this problem as an opportunity to try out a new medication, and a strategic therapist may plunge into the social context and how it serves to maintain the problem. A solution-focused therapist may ask the miracle question and zero in on strengths that can be amplified.

In standard talk therapy I may certainly employ some of the above, but if the person is requesting hypnosis I typically begin with a brief discussion on how being stuck resides primarily in one place, the unconscious. I then ask them if they are willing to undergo a step-wise procedure directed at perturbation and unconscious problem solving. If I get a green light I usually proceed with a story induction, standard deepening, and the Three Lessons story (Wallas, 1985; Gafner and Benson, 2000) whose meta-message is that people have resources within themselves to help solve their problems. Then, I continue with two or three sessions of ego-strengthening, which tests response and builds a foundation before commencing an exploratory and instigative intervention such as the above.

If these efforts are successful the client will report new behavior or a new way of viewing the problem, usually within two weeks. As a mechanism and its time frame, this is consistent with studies on paradoxical intervention and its outcome (Shoham-Salomon and Rosenthal, 1987). As a part of this process I typically set up finger signals for unconscious questioning. This involves responses for *yes*, *no*, and *I don't know/I am not ready to answer yet*, all on one hand. After the story I will then ask specific questions such as, "Tom, I want to ask a question of your unconscious mind and the question is this: 'Is guilt, yes, guilt, holding you back at this time?' Taking as much time as you need, you may answer with one of those fingers on your right hand."

I may also ask general questions using finger signals such as, "Tom, let your mind drift and dream ... and right now I want to direct a question to the back part of your mind. Is there anything else that comes to mind that can be of assistance to you at this time? Taking as much time as you need, you may answer with one of those fingers." Accordingly, the therapist accumulates new data both through unconscious questioning during the procedure and conscious verbal responding during the debriefing.

Acceptance

You may sit back and get comfortable in your own way and close your eyes if you wish as I share with you what I experienced one day. It was a beautiful summer morning in rural southern Illinois. After working for a couple of hours in my garden I rested on the porch. I sat back in the chair, leaned back and closed my eyes, and immediately entered a state of *deep reflection*. I certainly cannot recall everything from that morning but I do remember the complete and total *relaxation of my face*, and I remember how the words of my father appeared in my mind. "Don't be a slacker" entered and exited my gauzy consciousness. My jaw became slack, very loose was my face, and the rest of me was *detached*, as if my arms and legs belonged to another. I thought to myself, "Oh, may this wonderful feeling last forever," and my mind *drifted and dreamed*. I didn't even hear the delivery truck as it chugged up the driveway, nor did I see the person as she approached, even though my eyes were looking right at her. Do you *accept* this package?" she asked once, and then twice. My eyes finally focused on the FedEx driver and I hastily scribbled my name for the woman, who must have thought she had stumbled on a drugged individual way out in the country. She soon evaporated and I resumed my reverie.

It was highly curious how other things, negative things that I customarily told myself, were completely absent from my mind as I daydreamed amidst those captivating moments lost in time, it was such a delightful and eternal pace! I had heard the caw of crows in the woods before, but had never really listened and sensed the gentle breeze across my face, the chirping of birds, the whirring sound of approaching hummingbirds, but today all these sensations seemed a part of me, as I was completely absorbed in my surroundings. Absorbed yet detached, how wonderfully intriguing! However, with the cry of a distant loon a very small part of me awakened and I was reminded of the season of old roses, and that at one time, long ago, I had lost my ease.

I had many dreams, just like now as I write these words when the pen moves across paper of its own accord. The words flow from my daydream to the pen in my hand, a very heavy hand. My heart was once heavy. I remember when I was young and I played with my older sister's jack-in-the-box, turning the crank until it exploded from its hiding place, frightening me anew each and every time. Pushing it back inside was the difficult part for little hands. As an adult I continued to say to myself, "Isn't it my duty to push everything back inside?"

Many painful years later, with too much practice at pushing feelings back inside, a spiritual guide commented on my cycle of toxic emotion and its suppression. She said, "You don't look like a recycling center. Cans here, glass over there, paper products right down here. Maybe a toxic waste dump is more apt for you," she noted.

I let myself drift and dream again, body in slumber on the porch, knowing that serious thoughts are fully capable of entertaining themselves *over there* in the woods. I don't need to be part of their amusement. Yes, the forest with its many years of accumulated leaves composting on its floor, I can think of nothing more rich than that *humorous/humus* as a medium for growth, were only I the mental equivalent of such topsoil. Maybe one day. In the meantime I dreamed and drifted. Someone said to me once, "Let your experience deepen as I count down from 10 to 1, beginning now, 10, … 9, … 8, … just how deep can a person go? Always in the comfort of the driver's seat … 7, 6, 5, 4, 3, 2, and 1, that's the way," I can still hear her words. I know now what it means when they say, "My voice will go with you."

We have all *accepted* lesser things. Why not the same with bigger things? Someone might say to you, "Here is a tomato plant for your garden, or a loaf of bread I want to share with you." "Thanks, I'll try it," you might answer. I knew a boy named Frankie who had a balloon, a bright red one. He opened his hand and *let it go*, just *let it go* … I also knew a woman who came through a terrible event in one piece – physically at least – but she continued to be plagued by unwanted thoughts which she was unable to eliminate from her mind. Along the way she learned an invaluable mental trick, which was this: she *imagined*, just imagined, that she had a remote control in her hand and *turned down* the volume of those thoughts, yes, she *turned down* the volume until the thoughts were barely audible. But that has nothing to do with the FedEx package, which I didn't open until the next day.

I'll always remember my daydream that day on the porch and to this day I can bring it back whenever I sit back and *close my eyes*, just letting that feeling of total comfort take over both my mind and body. I deeply appreciate sharing this experience with you.

Notes for practice

For some clients, this induction will be too purposeful or didactic, others not. Notice how the deepening was inserted early on, something that you can experiment with as you tinker with the other inductions to suit your particular needs. Some key suggestions are underscored. I have had some clients in whose unconscious minds these suggestions percolated, later surfaced to the conscious mind, and initiated long overdue behavior change. For others, it led to their enrolling in an Acceptance and Commitment Therapy group. I'm always thinking pattern interruption and small steps. One therapist I knew had a pair of baby's shoes on his desk as a reminder. Misspeak is introduced in this induction. With this elegant indirect device the therapist appears to misspeak. The first word is the suggestion. It is quickly followed by the next word which, along with the rest of the sentence, serves to lead the person away from conscious analysis. In the last paragraph an eye closure is presented as a posthypnotic suggestion. Posthypnotic suggestion can also be incorporated in the anchor, or associational cue: "Please make for me now a little circle with your thumb and first finger, let those fingers touch … this is your anchor or reminder, when you need to slow down, take stock of things, something you always carry with you … I knew a woman one time who found herself making that little circle at work as well as at home …" By the second session *I always* build in an anchor. "It's a tool for your toolbox," I explain.

Begin to have your clients responding early in the process. Rehearsing the anchor is one way. Another way is with a head nod or deep breath. Maybe you're half way through an induction and you pause: " ... doing just fine, we're about half way through the trance induction process ... give yourself a few moments to let your experience develop, and when you're ready to proceed, let me know by nodding your head ..."

As *accept* is the meta-suggestion in this induction, you can set up the induction by seeding accept. It can be any variety of things, e.g., before you start, you comment, "I've *accepted* a lot of referrals lately, which is good," or, "I've come to *accept* all the traffic on the freeway." This seeds the target suggestion which is later activated when you mention it again. Read more on seeding in the glossary.

Kokopelli's Legs

As I read you the following account I would like you to sit back, close those eyes if you wish, and let yourself become immersed in a tale about the hunchbacked flute player. It was around 1985, I can't remember for sure. I found myself at a trading post on the Navajo Indian reservation.

I was *tired*, my *legs* were *heavy*, and I stopped to *yawn* as I exited the trading post — suggestions and started for the parking lot. I passed an elderly Indian man in a sweater and jeans who had been there when I went in. He sat there, *unmoving* and *expressionless*, and — catalepsy when I had gone some twenty paces I heard someone say, "Hey *there!*" I turned and said, "You speaking to me, sir?" "*In here, — apposition of opposites out there*, no one else is present, is *there*?" he responded in a soft, even voice. "Come *here*," he said. "What in the world for?" I asked, as I started toward him, suddenly surprised into alertness. "You'll soon *dis-* — suggestion *cover*," he answered as he rose to his feet.

I could now see he was a big man with long arms and legs who towered over me by a good 12 inches. *Normally* I would have been fluff more cautious with strangers but for some reason I followed him as he trudged slowly to a small building that stood in the shade of an ancient tree behind the trading post.

We left the bright afternoon sunshine and entered the darkened one-room structure. As my eyes adjusted to the low light I felt my shoes on the smooth pinewood floor far below, a stark contrast to the dusty high desert outside. Muted Native American flute music emanated from somewhere.

I could *not see* the man when he spoke again. negative hallucination "I saw the guided imagery bumper sticker on your car," he began, "and I think what I have in here may be of immeasurable interest to you. Please sit down in that recliner." I groped to my side, located the chair, and sat down. I immediately *sank deeply* into it suggestions and realized just how *tired* I was; but I also realized that I felt increasingly curious as well as trusting. "*What* in the world can be question going on here?" I wondered. "You'll *dis-* suggestion *cover* that momentarily," said the man. The words jolted me, but only for an instant as I had just then noticed images of Kokopelli, the Anasazi hunchbacked flute player. They were everywhere!

Kokopelli was woven into the wool rug on the floor. He was on the walls. He was in mobiles hanging from the ceiling. Copper, wood, plastic, big and small, turquoise blue, red, yellow … A dizzying assortment of Kokopellis, hundreds and hundreds of them enveloping me.

The man's *voice* again *penetrated* from with-   suggestion
out. "You may call me Curtis," he said be-
fore adding, "Tell me your name later." He
sat down near me. "I studied with the famous Dr. Milton Erickson in Phoenix in the
1970s. He called me his token red man, such
a delight was he, making puns, doing one
thing with his *right* hand, and another with   apposition of opposites
his *left*, which sometimes *left* you *wondering*   suggestion
just what was going on. I promised him I
would share my knowledge with others.
I remember his exact words: 'Red, my good
man, you *can't not* continue your develop-   double negative
ment, won't you?' That man firmly grasped
both my spirit and unconscious mind and
he holds on still," he said.

The lights dimmed further, the flute music
became louder, and I remember closing my
eyes, settling deeper into the chair. What
followed – I hesitate to say – may have actually occurred in fact, or may be a product
of my dream, I really don't know, but right
now, at this moment, I am recalling that
Curtis turned on one of those slide projec-
tors that they had in those days. I will now
try to recount my experience that followed.

"Dissociation may be the essence of trance,"   suggestion
he said, as I gazed at the images shown
by the projector, a whirl of petroglyphs
and pictographs, jumping deer, dancing
antelopes, bighorn sheep, coyotes, frogs,
lizards, feet here, *those* hands over there,   dissociative language
hands with six digits, seven, right ... and
above, below, in their midst, there he was,
the flute player, *lying down, standing up*, one   apposition of opposites
Kokopelli, many Kokopellis, in squares, cir-
cles, rectangles, *lighter*, then *darker*.

"*Disconnectedness* can lead to highly pleas- dissociation
ant and curious sensations," Curtis contin-
ued as another slide clicked into place. There
were more flute players, back hunched over
far, back bent slightly, back erect, back bent
over backwards, and back again were the
animals in motion, different colors, a swirl
of colors, a riot of colors, antelopes with
three legs, two, six, body here, leg over
there, frogs leaping, stick figures carrying
baskets, dried corn *drizzling down, floating* apposition of opposites
up. It was a most invigorating experience
and I saw my own *body floating*, above the dissociation
trading post, looking down, there was the
Grand Canyon. I was splashed by the cold
Colorado River.

There was Hopi First Mesa, Lake Powell,
Glen Canyon before Lake Powell, El Morro,
Newspaper Rock, White House Ruin, San
Cristobal, such breathtaking vistas from my
floating vantage point. I could see so far, I
saw *into the future*, myself in the future … age progression
And there he was again, playing the flute dissociation
with *no hands*. I heard, "Tha-a-t's the way."
It was gravelly and grandfatherly, the way
Erickson sounds on those old tapes. "*Sep-* suggestions
aration can lead to sleep in the extremities," intoned Curtis softly, and my *slumber*
deepened, as I *dreamed* and *drifted* for what
seemed like the *longest duration*. time distortion

My next conscious recollection was being in
my car, driving down the road, the trading
post was in the rearview mirror. The following year I returned to the trading post. I inquired about Curtis, but no one knew him.
The tree was there just as I remembered it,
but no building stood behind the trading
post. None of that seems to matter now because I can still hear the music and when
I close my eyes I can still hear his words.
Source: Young (1990).

Deepening

You may let your experience deepen as I tell you what happened to me one Saturday morning as I set out in my car. I drove for a while and then came to a sign that said yard sale. I peered at the sign through the windshield and drove on. After a short time I came to a sign that said rummage sale. I slowed down briefly and continued on. Soon, I encountered a sign that said garage sale. I nearly stopped but decided upon further exploration. In a few minutes I came to a sign that said estate sale. I pulled over, turned off the key, sat back, closed my eyes, took one very deep breath, and then drifted off into another state.

Notes for practice

In an induction, dissociation is a highly employable hypnotic phenomenon. It is a cardinal feature of trance and one that is useful, especially with people who normally dissociate, such as clients with post-traumatic stress disorder (PTSD). In debriefing with PTSD clients I often tell them that their experiencing dissociation in an induction is a good thing, as it builds on their natural ability to space out and feel disconnected. You may be wondering if such an approach might unwittingly lead to more pathological dissociation, and the answer is no. Instead, our employing this naturally-occurring – albeit pathological in the natural environment – phenomenon may best be framed as utilization, as it embraces what is problematic and builds on in the desired direction, which is therapeutic trance.

Notice in these inductions the liberal use of dissociative language to encourage dissociative feelings. I usually say *that* hand, not your hand, or *those* feet of yours *out there*, rather than your feet. Dissociative language, like any artifice, is good, but only up to a point. Too frequent mentioning of anything may only draw conscious attention to it, where our purpose is to stay beneath the radar.

A word on deepening and depth of trance. Most writers acknowledge that deeper trance is better than light, but that many clients in light trance can achieve benefit. Now, some current writers eschew the idea of depth in general, striving instead to develop associations *laterally*.

In the course of a conversation, or listening to music, countless associations are generated – all presumably lateral, but perhaps up or down or diagonal, if that is possible. Then, we have the trance experience in which the therapist's voice and words generate innumerable associations referenced as past, present, and future. Unless we stop the session and ask for a verbal report from the client every few seconds it is impossible to verify this as fact. The best we can do is ask for feedback in post-trancework discussion, or check with the client next time to learn new data. Now, if we're talking about *new resources* which, to me, is more useful than associations, then we should expect to see changes in the client subjectively, objectively, behaviorally, or on a paper-and-pencil measure.

4. Finding Your Own Voice

Finding Your Own Voice

Let's take a moment and compare the hypnotherapist to a general surgeon. The surgeon has operating room privileges, scalpels, saws and similar tools, ample assistance from an anesthesiologist and other personnel, and a license to write prescriptions for antibiotics, opiates, and other medications once the surgery is done. But hypnotherapists get the job done with only one thing: *their voice*.

To use a less sanguine metaphor, let's compare a radio announcer to a TV announcer. The latter has benefit of a host of visual aids, while radio announcers can influence their audience with only one thing: *their voice*. When I train therapists to do hypnosis I liken the therapist to the radio announcer. The radio announcer's audience is similar to our clients who are sitting there with their eyes closed. Your new perm, nicely trimmed beard, or the mouth wash you just gargled will have little or no influence with either audience, as they both care about only one thing: *your voice*. Therapists new to hypnosis often say things such as, "I don't like the sound of my voice." I say to them, "Well, then, let's practice. Hypnosis is like anything else. The more you practice, the better you get." People may practice in the shower or with a tape recorder. I know people who get the feel of a script by reading it to their spouse, or even their dog or cat. Some work on their hypnotic patter while stuck in traffic. It's all about practice. Remember Marilyn Monroe's squeaky girlish voice in those old movies? Well, I had an intern once, Kay, whose voice was just like Marilyn Monroe's. The very first day she said, "Just listen to my voice!" and "What would you do if you had a voice like mine?" I was stumped and thought, "Oh my, this is not good." But even Kay, through tedious practice with a tape recorder, succeeded in developing a fairly good hypnotic voice.

What is a good hypnotic voice?

Generally, a hypnotic voice will be melodic and smooth, and have less pitch and volume. Does this mean you should speak in a boring monotone? Sometimes. When clients tell me, "You have such a nice voice," I answer with, "Believe me, it took years of practice for me to become this boring!" I have my conversational voice, my therapist voice, and my *hypnotic voice*. Maybe you have more than three. A conversational voice may be breezy and carefree with little attention paid to enunciation. In other words, it is very casual, maybe even sloppy, and there's nothing wrong with that *except* when it carries over to your other voices. My therapist voice may be casual at times, but in speaking to clients I am careful to pronounce words completely and with sufficient volume. However, when I want to emphasize a point, I speak in a lower pitch and with less volume to lend emphasis to a key point. Then there's my *hypnotic voice*, which is probably the most varied.

People who have done hypnosis for a while come to appreciate the need for clear, careful enunciation, and speaking with the front part of the mouth, not strangling words in the throat. A psychologist friend of mine used to remind interns, "Massage 'em with your words." And that's precisely what I think about, a massage, as I'm speaking to clients in trance. I want my voice to be inviting, welcoming, and embracing. Milton Erickson told clients, "My voice will go with you." This is a valuable suggestion, but it is not likely to be a successful post-hypnotic suggestion unless your voice is a memorable one.

I often employ "my voice will go with you" but more indirectly: "From here on who knows if this voice can go with you?" or even more indirectly, "One woman one time imagined, just imagined, a voice accompanying her ..." Of course, it is even better to tie the suggestion to something that is likely to occur in the natural environment, e.g., "You may find my words to be an ally when you take one deep, satisfying breath."

Contrasts are your friend

It is believed that a subtle vocal alteration is a true unconscious suggestion. So, during trancework, I always speak with lower volume and decreased rate when I deliver a key suggestion: "and all those balloons, red ones, blue ones, green ones, *she just let them go*." As I am saying, "she just let them go" I am thinking "massage 'em with your words," but I am also imagining a gentle breeze blowing across the client's cheek, and a soft pulsing of words emanating from deep within the room. I typically begin a session speaking with a louder volume and then gradually lower it as I get into the induction. But I also toy with volume, rate, and pitch *throughout the session*. Contrast this variance with a slow, consistent monotone that never alters. That would make *me* bored and could put the person to sleep. It's hard enough to keep people awake these days with all the medications they take.

I believe that altering the qualities of our patter is in itself trance inducing in the same way that apposition of opposites is trance inducing, so, "I don't know if in your hands, or your feet, you'll begin to notice a coolness or warmth, heaviness or lightness, tingling or numbness ..." This juxtaposition of opposite hypnotic phenomena helps lull a person into trance. So, too, our alteration of volume, rate, and other qualities further hastens the process.

Your voice in an induction and other scripts

Many inductions, stories, anecdotes, techniques, and so on, I have memorized, but some things I simply can't remember and have to rely on reading scripts. Clients come to expect and appreciate reading to them as a natural part of the "stimulus control." When writers turn in a script for a movie or a play they generally include very few hints on how lines in the script should be delivered. Writers are confident that professional actors will bring their experience and intuition to bear on the written word. If the script calls for emphasis or certain feelings to be conveyed to the audience, writers leave it up to the actors to communicate the appropriate emotion. So, too, with a hypnosis script that I write. I might underscore a key suggestion, but aside from that, I trust that the reader will identify from the context when to speed up or slow down, and when to alter the quality of the voice to fit the clinical situation. For sure, ten different therapists may individualize the reading of an induction – or a story or anything else – in many different ways, and that is good. Just as it is desirable to tailor therapy in general to individuals and their particular situation, so, too, it is desirable to adapt your reading of an induction to both your particular client and how you are feeling on any given day.

I also hope that if you haven't already done so, with practice you will eventually be able to ad-lib certain material without having to read it. As you become more comfortable with an induction or story, it can become a part of your own repertoire. As you develop your hypnosis craft you can truly add your own voice by devising your own inductions, stories, and anecdotes. By not having to continually glance back and forth between script and client you will be in a better position to both pace ongoing behavior and adapt your voice to the ever-changing clinical scenario.

A few more notions

Check closely for hearing loss. If you have to shout, "JUST LET YOURSELF DRIFT OFF ...," well, you get the picture. Instead, use an audio amplifier. With mine, I speak into the small microphone in the hand-held amplifier whose cord is connected to headphones worn by the client. This can also help if you have a noisy hallway outside your office. Save your voice. One benefit of doing hypnosis is that you get to take a break from clients dumping negative affect into your ears. However, several hypnosis clients in one day may tax your voice. I counter this by employing ample pauses and using periods of silence as a deepening, both of which give me time to rest and collect my thoughts. I also occasionally have clients speak during trance, e.g., "Tell me now, with your words, what are you experiencing deep inside ..." Clients speaking during trance may lighten trance. After they speak I usually say something like, "Okay, take two deep breaths and let yourself sink even deeper."

Sit erect. If you are slouched, or if your legs are crossed, your breathing may be impeded. Notice your own breathing – breathe deeply and often as you reel out your patter. I keep in mind one image: a *column* of breath. I want to start every so often with a nice, column of breath. Also, I *always* have a drink of water within reach. Times that I've forgotten to do so I inevitably developed a cough or parched throat. Keep your hands away from your face. If you talk with your chin resting on your hand, or if you have a hand anywhere near your mouth, your voice will be partially blocked.

You *will* find your own voice, one that you are comfortable with, and it will serve you well. Practice different voices during day-to-day conversation, in therapy, or when you're alone. For therapists who are still unable to find their voice, I developed a story about Samuel Edgar, who, after much travail, succeeded in finding his voice (Gafner, 2004).

5. Guided Imagery Inductions

Guided Imagery Inductions

The Magic Theater

Let those eyes close now and allow yourself
to begin to appreciate the wonderful comfort that can develop when both your body
and your mind really *slow down*. No doubt   suggestions
you can recall other times in the past when
you *let go* and drifted off into another state,
not a state like Indiana or Texas, but a state
of mind where the deepest part of you was
open and *receptive* to new experience.

In a moment I will invite you to accompany me on a most interesting journey of discovery ... which can happen *all by itself*. For one person it might be letting go *effortlessly*, for another *freeing up* one's self, *independent* of conscious deliberation, and for someone else it just occurs *automatically*. "Mental *cruise control*" was how one woman put it. Effortless, independent, automatic, unconscious: they all may point in the direction trance. Going down a real road requires conscious attention, while none is required on this journey.

suggestion covering all possibilities

But first, I want your experience *to deepen* as I count backward, down from 20 to 1, 20, ... 19, ... 18, ...

deepening

(Client's name), imagine now, just imagine yourself in a building, any building you like, perhaps one you've been in before, a familiar place. There you are, on the first floor, walking down the hall, and you pass a door that you paid little attention to previously. You pause at the door and see that it is a service elevator. You touch a button that opens the door, you enter, and the door gently closes. You think to yourself, "Should I go up or down?" Of its *own accord* your hand extends out from your body and you touch the down button. The elevator descends rapidly and in a moment the door opens. You step out and gaze upon a small theater. It is the Magic Theater and you take a seat in the back row.

dissociation

It is very quiet in the theater and glancing around you see that you are alone. A profound *fatigue* comes over you, your eyes close all by themselves, and you enter a most pleasant *sleep*. In your sleep you

suggestion hypnotic dreaming

dream, drift and dream, for what seems like the *longest time*. In your dream the curtain time distortion on the stage opens and you see a movie screen. On the screen you see various nature scenes. One is Alpine Spring and you drink in the most inviting and peaceful setting you have ever seen. Then, your eyes move to the other scenes, one entitled Desert Solitude, another called River Raft Trip through the Grand Canyon, one a visit to a South Seas Island, and yet another entitled Canadian Wilderness.

Your eyes move back and forth from one to another. Each is most appealing, one more captivating than another. You then hear a woman's voice that says, "Select one and only one *now*." In your mind you choose Alpine Spring, and suddenly the whole screen fills with Alpine Spring. You see yourself standing beside a bubbling spring high in a lovely mountain wilderness. Is this Switzerland? Are you in the Himalayas? You do not know, and it really doesn't matter. The woman's voice is heard again, this time in a mere whisper. She says, "That's right, there's *nowhere* you need to be, *nothing* to not knowing / not doing think about, *no one* to please, *nothing* to do or change, all you have to do is just sit there and breathe."

The wildflower blossoms are yellow, some are white. Some in the distance are blue. Your eyes drink in a riot of color. The scents are most invigorating. The warm sun and refreshing mountain air envelop you. "I feel absolutely wonderful," you think to yourself.

"Your *journey begins,*" says the voice one   suggestion
more time, and you begin to walk down the
trail. The scents you experience, the sounds,
the breathtaking vistas, all are of such indescribable clarity. There is a spring in your
step as you move along briskly, confidently,
occasionally stopping to appreciate something that holds you in its embrace. Has a
minute passed, or several *hours*? You do not   time distortion
know, and it is of no import whatsoever.
Never before have you known such *comfort*   suggestion
and well-being.

The voice appears again. That voice is out
there, but it is as if it reverberates from deep
within you. It says, "In a moment you will   suggestion
experience something most meaningful to
you. *Will it be* an evergreen epiphany?" "A   question
what?" you ask yourself. "An epiphany of
any hue would be most welcome indeed!"
you think. You wish the voice would speak
to you again. All is now very quiet, inside
and outside. You continue on the trail for
what may be a short time or a long *duration,*
you have no way of determining *time,* clock   time distortion
time, time on a calendar, *seconds* or *hours*
within a dream. In your dream you speak
to yourself: "Why can't this last forever?"
are the words.

You know that you can *come back* to Alpine   posthypnotic
Spring any time you want, simply by clos-   suggestion
ing your eyes. There is a mountain goat in
the distance. It is *unmoving,* as of *stone,* its   catalepsy
gaze on you is unwavering. These lovely
flowers by my feet, what are they called?
Color, texture, and meaning tumble in your
mind. Pine trees in the distance, moss by
your feet. Shades of green about you and
deep inside yourself. Blue sky in the distance deepens your reverie.

You continue your journey. *Isn't it* high- question
ly curious what percolates deep within?
(Pause for several seconds.) Your eyes
open. You are back in the theater, the curtain on stage is closed and you arise from
your seat, *woodenly* at first, as you make catalepsy
your way back to the elevator.
Source: Young (2007).

Second deepening

I will be quiet for a few minutes while your unconscious mind
contemplates today's experience. During this deepening, who
knows what else will surface from deep within.

Notes for practice

Normally we offer clients a deepening only one time, *after* the
induction; however, in this case it was inserted early on to absorb, and then again at the end to foster further unconscious
search. There are many ways you can structure your sessions.
By now you may be starting to see what might work for you.
An induction such as Magic Theater usually elicits new or different unconscious responses, thus producing newfound resources that can be integrated during the debriefing. As such,
your therapy goal of exploration may be met with the induction alone. Sometimes I will tell a story as the therapy component following The Magic Theater. I have found, though, that
in some cases a story leads them sufficiently away from material discovered during the induction so that it is forgotten by
the time you get to realerting. This isn't good if you were eager
to discuss it; however, for many clients, their discoveries may
surface again when they close their eyes. For posthypnotic
suggestion, most writers advocate something that is likely to
occur in the natural environment. Erickson would use "when
you see a flash of light." I believe oftentimes you can access

this same process – albeit with conscious instigation – when clients practice relaxation by using their anchor.

The Forest

You can sit back and close your eyes, if you wish, as we begin this guided experience. First, I would like you to imagine, just *imagine*, a feeling of profound and soothing comfort beginning down at the soles of your feet. I don't know if that image of comfort is warm or cool, liquid or solid, abstract or literal, but it can be anything at all, and whatever it is, just let it happen now, going up your body, slowly or rapidly, up one leg first, or up both legs at the same time. That's the way, just let it happen …

Now, I don't know, and you may not either, just how long it will take for that pleasant feeling to reach the top of your head, seconds or minutes, but just let it happen of its own accord, as I continue to read to you.

It is a warm, sunny day and you find yourself in a beautiful forest. You've been here before, and you know it is a safe place. You feel absolutely *wonderful* as you start down a path on this journey of discovery. You walk for a couple of minutes, stop, and reach into your right pocket. You open the folded piece of paper which says, "Count down now, in your mind, from 10 to 1," that's the way, sinking deeper and deeper into a most delightful sense of relaxation. You place the paper in your left pocket and continue down the path, anticipating the joy of discovery that lies just ahead.

Your pace is brisk as you penetrate deeper and deeper into the forest, and you marvel at your newfound depth of relaxation, comfort, and well-being. You feel the life of the forest, the scents and sounds, and it is indeed a most remarkable experience. You stop, reach once again into your right pocket, and extract a typewritten page. You sit down, unfold it and begin to read.

One day not long ago a woman, well into her eighties, described a dream, yes, a dream. Most curiously I had the same dream beginning in my forties, and even now when I experience this dream I feel a certain disquiet, but also an odd comfort. Madge – her name is Madge – has passed on, but I'm glad I recorded what she told me about her recurrent dream.

Now, Madge's husband was in World War II, and she said, "He never told me the specifics of those two weeks on Iwo Jima. However, I relived Iwo Jima every day until my husband left this earth on Armistice Day in 1984.

"My doctor told me to walk down this same path, and one day I did so. When I reached into my right pocket the first time, the paper said one word, *courage*. I placed the paper in my left pocket and continued on down the path. After what seemed like the longest time I reached in my pocket again. The paper this time said two words, *loyalty* and *duty*. I crinkled up the paper and put it away. I continued down the path. My legs were heavy but my mind felt a curious levity."

The typewritten page ended. But your journey, kind listener, continues. You resume walking down the path. A crunching sound beneath your feet alerts you to small stones in the path. You stop, breathe deeply, and reach into your pocket one more time. The paper you extract has one word on it. That word is *love*.

You continue on, your feet propelling themselves forward. There is a fork in the path and without hesitation you turn down the right path. Your mind drifts and dreams, and something of indescribable clarity penetrates your consciousness. The joy of discovery provides you with an immeasurable comfort. The path is now nearing its end. Words resound in your head, and those words say, "I must take something with me to remember this day." What comes to mind is a complete surprise, a gift from today's experience. (Pause.)

And beginning now, I would like you to let yourself resume your normal, alert, waking state as I count from 1 up to 5, beginning to count now, 1, 2 ...

Notes for practice

You may wish to add a deepening before the realerting. I didn't think it was necessary as I was writing this induction. Remember, a deepening can be like others presented in this book, and it can also be a brief story, or anecdote, or something else that intuition dictates. Also, a guided imagery induction invites active verbal processing immediately afterward, as opposed to some material which you may wish to allow to percolate in the unconscious and discuss later. See what fits for you and your client.

Let's discuss something that can enhance both your effectiveness with hypnosis and the foregoing induction: *interspersal.* This technique is one of the many gifts bequeathed to us by Milton H. Erickson. Interspersal can be a brief anecdote inserted during an induction, deepening, or story, or even during a technique, such as age regression. It can also be a word or phrase inserted during one of those phases. The operative word is *insert.* I think to myself, "What does the client need to hear right now in order to improve?" and then I insert that key suggestion. Once or twice is usually sufficient in a session. If "let go" or "be strong" is what they need to hear, I intersperse it in the above induction, and with a subtle vocal shift.

Try it out. Use your intuition. Deviate from the script. Step out of your comfort zone. If you've never done this, it may sound oblique – and it is – but that's what's good about it because it helps you depart from the pro forma. You take this first step and you're immediately on the path to ad-libbing and developing your own material. When Erickson started out he wrote out every word in the induction long hand. His first efforts were thirty pages long. He gradually boiled it down to ten pages, and soon he didn't need to read anything. I would be proud if one day you don't even need to consult this book. When you do talk therapy you don't need a script. In hypnosis, you probably already have your own voice. You can also develop your own technique. That's the art of hypnosis.

Complex Canopies

Sit back, let your eyes close, and begin to go deep inside, because in a moment I'm going to ask you to suspend judgment and critical evaluation. Yes, I'm going to invite you on a highly imaginary experience. I'm going to lead you on a journey inside a tree, yes, deep within a tree. Please take a couple of nice, deep, relaxing breaths now before we begin ...

You have been traveling in the western United States and now you find yourself in northern California. It is now midday. You have always wanted to stand among the giant redwoods, no one else is around, and here you are now, amidst trees as tall as a thirty-five-story skyscraper. In this shady community of titans hazy shafts of sunlight illuminate your cozy natural chamber. The soil is firm beneath your feet. Your eyes blink once, twice, and then gently close, as your journey begins.

You wish to reach what is called the complex canopy and kiss the sky way above. High up there in these most ancient trees whose crowns host entire ecosystems. The wandering salamander spends its entire life span on top of that world. Scientists know why the redwood grows so tall, but one thing they don't know: *What keeps them from growing even taller?* Your task is to discover this mystery. However, you also have something inside of you that is puzzling, your own mystery that has remained just outside of conscious awareness for a long, long time ...

Your eyes open briefly, you gaze around, and you ask yourself, "How might I solve these two mysteries? I can't possibly climb up to the top and there is no conveyance to take me there." You breathe deeply and feel those eyes close again, and a few seconds later you have your answer. The ground beneath you disappears as you dissolve into a mist. How astounding to realize you have shrunk into a mere vapor, tinier than the head of a pin. You are then further distracted by a strong downward pull as you penetrate the soil. Soon you are deep within the ground beneath the ancient redwoods.

You feel both peaceful and energized as you enter the massive root system of a tree, and you begin to rise within the tree, slowly, steadily, assisted by the capillary action of the tree. You hear a voice, a disembodied voice, an auditory specter. Is it in here? Out there? It is a voice you have heard before, a voice that rises in pitch as if asking a question. It is now barely discernible and you strain to hear it, as you continue to rise, up, up, within the tree.

You are one with this tree, rising, rising within it. You have lost track of time, not knowing if you have been within this tree for moments or years. Again, a voice, your own voice, reverberates within you, or is it penetrating from without? "Why am I doing this?" asks the voice, which soon fades away. You continue to rise within and your experience becomes more profound, lighter in body, heavier and deeper in mind and spirit, a transcending experience, as your former world is left far, far behind ...

You recall previous experiences, lost in something pleasant, like a poem, or wonderful music, where seconds blended into minutes into hours, when time, time on a clock, on a calendar, did not matter in the least. Last year you attended a lecture on redwoods where someone said that the tallest trees grow along major streams on California's coast, where rich soils provide year-round moisture. The person said, "Remember, redwoods absorb water through the leaves – they love fog and rain – but most moisture comes from the soil."

You have in your experience other journeys, journeys in fact or journeys in mind, roads taken and roads avoided, dangerous ventures as well as safe ones. Today's journey is risky only in that you may receive answers to questions best not asked, and all that can be forgotten beginning now, as *discovery* awaits at the top. Fog, rain, and soil are distant entities as you continue your ascent, higher and higher, and your mental immersion deepens. Time past, time present, future time, all time is obscured and irretrievably lost amidst then-now-before-and-when? A thumping sound, is it in your chest or elsewhere? "How high have I come?" you ask yourself. You have no way of knowing if you have ascended a few inches or halfway up the tree. Which tree, the one you were standing closest to? How can you be doing this?

You reflect on your life, your satisfactions and regrets, failures and triumphs, yes, your satisfactions glow within you in this timeless void, and then you feel yourself constrict further as you are pulled up, up, and up. You suddenly emerge at the top. You are at the apex of the canopy. You grasp a branch with one hand, and with the other, you examine your body. You have returned to your normal size. You drink in the breathtaking vista as you cling to the branches. The breeze … you are swaying. It is so bright up here. The salamander eyes you curiously. You cling to a branch. In a nanosecond you are back on the ground and all is quiet. (Pause.) From your experience within the tree you have absolutely no idea what limits the redwood's growth. As for that other mystery, the mystery about yourself, an answer will be forthcoming shortly. But first, the groceries! You remember some groceries in the trunk of your car.
Source: Marquis (2006).

Notes for practice

This ends abruptly with a distraction to lead clients away from analysis. Instead, you may wish to omit that, include a deepening, and add a therapy component. I usually use this induction as is, stop after the induction, and ask clients to discuss it next time. Who knows what discovery will surface between sessions? I put this induction last among guided imagery inductions because it is rather bizarre, definitely not for everyone, especially claustrophobics! Then, who might appreciate Complex Canopies? Well, did you ever have to buy a gift "for the person who has everything"? So, this might be apt for the well-traveled client, or one who wishes exploration in a new and different way. As such, it is something like the ambiguous function assignment in talk therapy. It is good for someone who is "stuck." I ask the person ahead of time, "Say, I have this unusual guided imagery induction where you are inside of a tree, okay if we try that one today?"

6. Confusional Inductions

Confusional Inductions

Just Forget about Amnesia

You may sit back and close your eyes, if you wish, as we begin today's relaxation experience as I read you the following.

Someone in the Lankton Institute in Switzerland said one time, "We've had several people come to the clinic who *wanted* to relax, let go, and journey in a meaningful way to somewhere else, but they weren't able to do so for precisely one reason: unconscious resistance. In other words the back part of their mind was working against them. "I want to let go, but I just can't experience amnesia," was what they typically reported. Accordingly, the following induction was devised by one of the Lankton consultants to help these folks achieve the presumably unattainable. Hopefully what follows will permit mental absorption to a mild degree, allow an arresting of attention to a moderate degree, or yield an interruption of the conscious set, or suspension of critical reasoning to at least a moderate extent, thus reserving an even deeper trance for another occasion. This was read to one person one time who gleefully remarked afterward, "I don't know how you did it, but thanks for captivating me in a most enjoyable experience." That person, I recall, was especially adept at activating listening with the third ear.

"Last time I went into trance I think I remembered everything," said Edith, who at the time was being attended to by Dr Lankton himself, who answered, "Amnesia? Just forget amnesia, Edith, especially amnesia with spontaneous recollection, that only occurs in less than 30% of cases, and at this moment I have no way of knowing if you are among the 29%, 51%, 48%, 58%, or even 68%, something that can easily be obfuscated among other numbers like date of birth, address, winning lottery number, high/low temperature of the day, or other numbers, mere digits that they are, but digits in hands or feet may be of greater import than something that can slip the mind."

Lankton continued, "Listen closely, Edith, to the following numbers, as I will ask you to recall them in approximately 360 seconds or less. Close those eyes and concentrate on the following: 548, 1027F, 3, 720, 9333, 10R, 22, 43, 777G, 6, 7, 348E, 4, 11, and 2501T." Edith carefully mulled over each number as it was received, registering them carefully in her mind. Lankton sat back, took a sip of water as he thought, "I always forget how parched those numbers make me." He observed Edith, whose eyes had closed, but her eyelids were fluttering as if *something was going on* deep inside. Lankton was taken aback as Edith muttered, "How is anyone supposed to remember all those numbers?"

"Any one, any two, don't preoccupy yourself with any of that, ma'am, as amnesia is our topic today and a useful byproduct in your case may be the most enjoyable of trance experiences which, in itself, is very worthwhile, something quite easily forgotten," he noted. Just then Edith appeared to sink deeper into her chair, her body heavy and unmoving. Later, when she was awakened Edith would report, "My body was here and out there at the same time my mind was somewhere else, if you know what I mean."

Lankton's own eyes had closed, his right arm had grown extremely light and his hand had levitated of its own accord, floating out in front of him. The doctor had for the time ceased paying attention to his subject, having become absorbed in his own reverie. Several seconds passed, perhaps a minute or two, it is not known for sure, and then Lankton said, "Edith, often I try to recall *something* – where I left my keys, whether or not I locked a door – and the harder I try to remember, the farther away I am from recalling it ... *But* if I think of something else – the clouds in the sky, the traffic in the next lane – suddenly the memory surfaces in my conscious mind. That seems to happen all the time. Percolation isn't just for coffee pots, you know."

"720, 548, 2501T," muttered Edith. "Very good, you're on the right track. But right now let's occupy the front part of your mind with the following so the back part of your mind can continue to solve the problem," said the doctor. "Breathing in, in your mind, a color, any color will do. A luxuriant lavender, a regal gold, do that now, in your imagination, Edith, that's right ... and exhaling another color, perhaps a verdant green, a bright orange ... breathing in a color, breathing out a color ..."

Edith's breathing had become profoundly regular ... even ... comfortable, as she drifted and dreamed. An uncertain interval of time passed. Lankton's arm had by now descended to his lap. After several more seconds Lankton spoke again. "Isn't it intriguing how your extremities can at once feel tingling-lightness-warmth-numbness-heaviness-coolness-detachment? Or marked curiosity or comfort elsewhere in the body? While your mind, yes, that mind ..."

The doctor then asked Edith to recite those numbers – backwards – and she did so quite easily, something the good doctor had witnessed only once previously in forty-three years at the Institute.

Notes for practice

No deepening here? Well, try one from another induction, or even better, devise your own. Let's recall the law of parsimony: do only what is necessary to achieve the desired effect. Applying that to inductions, on one extreme, we have the well-practiced client who needs very little direction to go into trance: "Just sit back, close your eyes … and when you're sufficiently deep in order to do the work you need to do today, your *yes* finger will rise." Save your breath, it's not needed. In the vast middle are those folks who require some guidance achieving trance. For them, a story or guided imagery induction does the job. About 10% of the U.S. population is considered non-hypnotizable. I estimate that we can cut that figure to 5% by using a confusional induction. If they fail to respond to other inductions, they often will go into trance with a confusional one, and once they do, you normally can return to a story or guided imagery induction, as you've broken through the unconscious resistance. In rare cases I continue with confusion.

West is Right

You may sit back and close those eyes if you wish, as I read you an induction called West is Right. To be sure, if you look at most maps east is to the right and west is on the left, and that may give you a little hint of what is to follow, as my purpose here is quite singular: to get in beneath the radar in order to permit you to let go and experience trance in any way you choose. I would like you to try to follow this story as best you can, even though it is designed so that most people's conscious minds *won't* be able to make sense of it, and all the while their unconscious minds are freed up to amuse themselves in their own unique way.

Now, to begin, I would like you to take a couple of nice, deep breaths, and just let yourself sink into that chair. By the time we're done today it may seem like many minutes have passed while in reality very few minutes of clock time have elapsed. Or, on the other hand, it may seem that this process has gone by quite rapidly, zooming by in a very few minutes, while in fact quite a long period of time has gone by. And it really doesn't matter, because there's absolutely nothing at all that you need to know, or do, or think about. There's nowhere you need to be, no one to please, no expectations to meet, and all you really need to do is just sit there and breathe, letting the words drift in and drift out.

I would like you to imagine, just imagine, that you are gazing at a map of a city. The name of the city isn't important, but the map is indeed important. This street map shows Central Avenue as the east–west dividing line. Streets to the east of Central are named for U.S. states – California, Wyoming, Montana, Utah, and Arizona. The streets west of Central are similarly named – Maryland, Connecticut, New York, Maine, and Rhode Island. Broadway Boulevard is the south–north dividing line. Streets north of Broadway are named South Carolina, Florida, Georgia, Louisiana, and Tennessee.

Sarah Inskeep was a driver for the Checker Cab Company in this small city, population less than 20,000. She had been on the job only two days and was having difficulty learning the streets and the locations of the various businesses. Her first passenger of the day got in at eight o'clock on Saturday morning. "I'm looking for a store called Slumberland," he announced. "Step on it, I'm in a hurry." Sarah called the dispatcher, who was away from the microphone. The man in back said, "I'll tell you where it is, just listen to me." Sarah nonchalantly pulled away from the curb. "Are you *listening* to me?" yelled the man. Sarah nodded in the affirmative. "Oh, it will be good to get rid of this guy," she thought.

His volume did not ease: "Cross Georgia, one-half mile up ahead, and go east on North Carolina for three blocks, and then hang a right on Montana for two miles, you're now heading south, and the address is 506 East Wisconsin. Got it?" Sarah accelerated. Traffic was light this Saturday morning. She drove on to Wisconsin and braked hard in front of 506 East, which was a vacant lot. The man continued, "You obviously weren't listening. Repeat my instructions back to me, but in reverse order." She answered, "From 506 East Wisconsin go north, hang a left on Montana after two miles, go west on North Carolina for three blocks, and then cross Georgia one-half mile up ahead."

"Very good," said the man, "however, I think I meant 510 West Maine. Remember this now: the streets south of Central are Wisconsin, Michigan, Iowa, and Minnesota; west of Broadway they are Maryland, New York, Connecticut, Maine, and Rhode Island; north of Central they are Georgia, Florida, South Carolina, North Carolina, and Louisiana; and east of Broadway they are California, Wyoming, Montana, Utah, and Arizona. Have you ever been to Maine in the fall?" Sarah didn't answer.

He continued even louder, "California is equidistant from Maryland, as is Utah from Maine, and Minnesota from North Carolina." Sarah pulled over opposite the town square. She gazed up at the big clock and thought about the *Back to the Future* movie and asked herself to which hand on the clock the mad scientist attached the wire. "There's the Chamber of Commerce," said the man, "I'll see if they're open on Saturday. They'll know where Slumberland is. Keep the meter running."

It seemed like the man was gone for the longest time. She put in a CD, sat back, closed her eyes, and listened to the words which after some pleasant flute music said, "I was accustomed to rushing through life, and I didn't slow down and rest, even in my sleep. Until one day, while climbing on a mountain trail near my home, when I met a very wise, elderly man. He took me aside and in a few minutes taught me the rest step, yes, the *rest step*. He told me, 'You can *rest* ever so briefly, ever so slightly, with each step you take,' and I began to apply this *rest step* in all aspects of my life.

"Just sit back now and let some pleasant experience from the past fill your mind. I don't know if that experience is walking along the beach, lying in bed at home, being absorbed in some pleasurable activity like listening to music or watching a movie … (pause), but let that happen now as I continue to talk to you about really slowing down your mind and your body both, and at intervals I will whisper, 'rest step,' and you will know exactly what this means. That's the way, just letting it happen all by itself, independently, autonomously, effortlessly, all by itself, no conscious effort at all is required.

"I went for a walk one time. It was so very pleasant walking in the park. No one else was present and any sound of traffic seemed far, far away. There was a large tree across the grassy expanse where I walked, and something about that big tree drew me to it ... *rest step.* (Pause.) I paced slowly and my legs felt light and springy as my eyes were focused on that tree. I remember that it was a warm day and no doubt there were clouds in the sky, but when your mind totally zeroes in on something, like a pleasant thought, a familiar song, or even the spring in your step, well, the rest of the world is excluded as your feet continue on down the walk."
Source: Powers (2006).

Notes for Practice

Many confusional inductions (Gafner and Benson, 2000) offer a high octane, non-stop barrage of confusion that is impossible for analytical "left brain" people to follow, e.g., "She was trying to find something and knew it was two rights and one left ... she took a left, a right, and another left; then a right, a left, another right, and was left without finding it, so she did a right-left-right combination followed by ... " and it goes on for a while, building the confusion and frustration so that the listener welcomes the opportunity to eventually escape from it – into welcome words of relaxation.

With West is Right only a modicum of confusion is offered, along with a dose of just plain aggravation which, like distraction, can also serve to overload. The client wishes to escape from this cognitive overload, and you offer him an exit in the desired direction, which is trance. I don't just spring a confusional induction on a client. Instead, I say, "We're going to try a little experiment today, something that might not make sense to you rationally, but which is something that can get in beneath the radar." You always want to be respectful, never let them think you're having fun at their expense. Lest we regard confusion as a bizarre or extravagant device, let's remember Erickson's words: "Confusion is the basis of most of my approaches to trance induction" (Rossi, 1982: 133). Lest we become enamored of any technique, I also keep in mind the words of Jeff Zeig (personal communication, 1999): "What's paramount is the client's response. Let that response be your guide, not the cleverness of the technique."

7. Afterword

Afterword

A few caveats

I wish I could say to you, "Now that you've read this book you can go out there, use these inductions with your clients, and everybody will love you for it." Certainly if you're in a private practice or work in a broad-minded agency this may be true. However, in other settings, such as in agencies where many of you are probably employed, you may need to educate people about hypnosis in order to pave the way for its acceptance. When interns complete training with me and go out into the world they are usually eager to begin to use their new skills on the job. But I warn them, "Remember, in some parts hypnosis is still a dirty word, so when you start to work at an agency, don't make yourself a target. Test the waters first by calling it relaxation therapy, ego-strengthening therapy, or something similar. If you have to field defensive questions like, 'Is this really hypnosis?' of course, you say it is." I also tell them to be prepared for questions like, "Do you have a license to practice hypnosis?"

We also discuss how others at the agency *won't* be asked the same questions, e.g., those practicing interactive guided imagery or mindfulness meditation. Instead, they may be asked if they've had training in those modalities, and hopefully they've had such training, just as you need requisite training in hypnosis. My point is that hypnosis has always carried baggage and hopefully one day it will not. When I am asked such questions, I patiently explain that I have no license to practice hypnosis nor does anyone. I don't have a license to do eye movement desensitization therapy or cognitive behavioral therapy or group anger management. I am a licensed clinical social worker and among the modalities I practice is hypnosis. I add that I am a member of the American Society of Clinical Hypnosis (ASCH) from which I have received – and provided – training, and the same goes for the Milton H. Erickson Foundation. So, prepare yourself with reading and training, but also be prepared for guarded inquiries.

Clinical privileges and practice guidelines

In your role at your agency you may need to draft a statement describing your "clinical privileges" to practice hypnosis. Agencies are always afraid of lawsuits and want to protect themselves so you need to be aware of this. Also, be prepared for your employer to say, "But there's no one here to supervise your hypnosis," so have a plan for that. Hopefully your colleagues or supervisor will be supportive, but in my experience, that is the exception, especially for master's level practitioners. At the time of writing there is discussion within ASCH to open up membership to bachelor's level folks; however, in general, at this time I support hypnosis practice only for master's level and above clinicians.

In addition to preparing yourself with regular training and supervision, one major thing you can do, especially early on in your practice, is to have a specific plan to practice only certain techniques with your client population. This may include say, for mood and anxiety disorders, limiting your hypnosis to inductions, deepenings, ego-strengthening stories, and building in an anchor to cue relaxation away from the office. Or, with chronic pain clients, certain inductions, deepenings, stories, and pain management techniques. Limiting yourself in these ways affords you a wide range of possibilities that still fall into "evidence-based practice." If you market your hypnosis *as adjunct*, as I do, then what you do hypnotically is a supplement to talk therapy. Billing yourself solely as a "hypnotherapist" is both unrealistic and limiting, as it implies that all you do is hypnosis for all clinical problems. Even in sessions consisting primarily of hypnosis you need to discuss various things so that the person's hypnotic experience is integrated. Also, many times I have had a plan to do hypnosis in a particular session but because of a crisis or other circumstances the session turned into supportive talk therapy instead.

Corrective and abreactive techniques

Another thing you can do to make your practice more acceptable to an employer is to avoid, especially early on, corrective or abreactive techniques. Both age regression and age progression are valuable techniques to master. However, when we *say* age regression many people *hear* past lives regression, and to some age progression connotes something out of science fiction. So, go easy with those techniques. Other useful interventions like smart window, amplifying the metaphor, and age regression, abreaction, and reframing, all wonderful techniques, may be viewed by others as exotic and mysterious – therefore, potentially *dangerous* – so don't even go there early on.

Inductions, deepenings, stories, and anecdotes fall within the realm of skill and self-efficacy building, whereas techniques like amplifying the metaphor are a clear departure in that their purpose is to effect a pattern interruption of the problem. Also, with many of these techniques, by design the client is encouraged to re-experience strong emotions during trance. Your mystified supervisor may then say, "But I thought hypnosis was supposed to be pleasant and relaxing!" Such techniques not only require a higher therapist skill level but also may result in temporary emotional upset by the client. So, in general I recommend that you refrain from corrective or abreactive measures until you're on firmer ground.

In summary

You have limitless tools in your hypnosis toolbox when you think of the tremendous range of inductions, deepenings, stories, anecdotes, and interspersal, which was discussed previously. You also have hypnotic techniques employed without formal hypnosis but within standard talk therapy. For years in the Veterans Affairs I had two concurrent anger management groups and at the conclusion of each session one of us would tell a brief Ericksonian-type story in which a mindfulness principle was embedded. Participants would say, "I know the point of that story!" and we would answer, "No, let's wait until next week and we'll discuss it." That way, unconscious processing could proceed without conscious interference. Of course, all group therapies can be augmented by stories. I regularly employ hypnotic language, such as truisms and apposition of opposites, as part of talk therapy, and nearly every session I throw in a story or anecdote – techniques that are unconscious communications. Clients become accustomed to my adding, "Let me tell you a little story about someone else who had a problem much like yours, and here's what they did ..."

Appendix I – A Compilation of Techniques

Compilation of techniques and decision tree

Remember the light bulb joke? In it, you are asked, "How many therapists does it take to change a light bulb?" The answer is ten. One to change the bulb and nine to tell stories about how Erickson would have done it better. (Gilligan, 1987). With that in mind, I present the following compilation of techniques. There are no doubt countless therapists who have innumerable ways of changing the light bulb, and the following is but one seasoned practitioner's attempt at doing so.

This is limited to five main problem areas in adults: anxiety disorders, chronic pain, insomnia, ego-strengthening, and unconscious exploration. For techniques with children, go to Mills and Crowley (1986) and Gafner and Benson (2003), to mention but a few resources.

Anxiety disorders

- Employing hypnotic phenomena – time distortion, dissociation, catalepsy, etc., e.g., for anxiety about being in an MRI machine, time in there slows down; imagining nervousness in the next room, imagining anxiety slowing down like molasses, etc. (Edgette and Edgette, 1995).

- Pattern interruption – disrupting or interrupting one or more aspects of the problem, typically the frequency, intensity, location, timing, or some other aspect (Cade and O'Hanlon, 1993).

- The following are from Hammond (1990):
    - Amplifying the metaphor technique
    - Pile of Rocks technique
    - Age regression, abreaction, and reframing technique
    - Smart Window technique
    - Slow Leak abreaction technique
    - Fractionated abreaction technique
    - Hypnotic Dreaming technique (alter aspects of dream)
    - Scab and Healing metaphor
    - Age progression technique
    - Collagen metaphor
    - Private Refuge metaphor
    - Island of Serenity metaphor
    - The Pool metaphor
    - Autogenic Rag Doll technique
    - Rational Emotive Behavior Therapy (REBT) technique
    - Various scripts for phobia

- The Door of Forgiveness technique
- Dumping the Rubbish technique
- Red Balloon metaphor
- Gandor's Garden technique
- Meeting an Inner Advisor technique
- Reframing dreams
- Corporate Headquarters of the Mind technique
- Time Distortion with Stop Watch technique.

- Reciprocal Inhibition technique – pair relaxation or positive image with fear to de-condition fear; for lack of self-confidence, for example, imaginally superimpose confident person image on fearful person image (Lankton and Lankton, 1983).

- Externally oriented self-hypnosis technique (Dolan, 1991).

- Dissociated containment technique (Dolan, 1991).

- Associational cues for comfort and security technique (Dolan, 1991).

Ego-strengthening

- Story (Gafner and Benson, 2003)

- Ego-strengthening anecdotes (Gafner, 2004)

- Story within a story (Gafner and Benson, 2003)

- Alternating stories (Gafner and Benson, 2003)

- Short burst technique (Personal Communication, Geary, 1999)

- The following are from Hammond (1990):

    - Barnett's Yes-Set method

- Ego-enhancement, five-step approach
- Suggestions for modifying perfectionism
- Helen Watkins's suggestions for self-esteem
- Serenity Place metaphor
- An Abstract technique for ego-strengthening
- Ugly Duckling metaphor
- Prominent Tree metaphor
- Fairy tales
- Fostering amnesia.

Chronic pain

As chronic pain may encompass a wide range of medical disorders, the client should have appropriate medical evaluation before beginning treatment. Hypnotherapy is usually adjunctive to cognitive behavioral therapy, individual, or group therapy, in addition to medical treatment. Secondary gain, guilt, blame, co-occurring psychological disorders, relational issues, or the compounding problems of advancing age can make chronic pain a complex and challenging clinical problem. Barber's (1996) *Hypnosis and Suggestion in the Treatment of Pain* is recommended reading.

- Interspersal technique (Rossi, 1980).

- Unconscious task technique – I use this most often for chronic pain. After induction and deepening, "Beginning now, I want to assign a job to the back part of your mind, and that task is this: full and complete comfort and relaxation in your body, and this can happen all by itself, effortlessly and independently, without any conscious effort, while I direct some words at the front part of your mind." Then tell a story.

- Full Comfort technique – "I want you to imagine a feeling of comfort beginning at the top of your head (or down at your feet), and I don't know if that feeling is coolness, warmth, or something else … and let that feeling descend down (or go up) your body now, just a bit at a time, and when that feeling has reached the soles of your feet (or top of your head), let me know by …" Follow with a story.

- Dial down the pain (Gafner and Benson, 2003).

- The following are from Barber (1996):

  - Gradual diminution
  - Glove anesthesia
  - Transforming the symptom/sensory substitution/alteration of sensation
  - Dissociation
  - Distraction
  - Displacement.

- The following are from Hammond (1990):

  - Age regression (for past mastery/competence, etc.)
  - Age progression (imagining future periods of comfort, imagine using anchor, etc.)
  - Suggestions for headaches
  - Melting Butter metaphor
  - Inner Advisor technique
  - Mystical States technique
  - Sympathetic Listener technique
  - Disorientation technique
  - Truisms for Developing Anesthesia technique.

Insomnia

Remember: much insomnia is secondary to un/under-treated depression or chronic pain.

- The following are from Gafner (2006):

  - Sound Sleep induction

- Boredom induction
- Slumber Pill induction
- Rumination induction
- Walking through Time induction
- Decline of Coral Reefs induction
- Forest of Stone induction
- Suggestions for improved sleep.

Unconscious exploration

- Age progression, age regression

- Automatic writing

- Automatic drawing

- Imaginary chalk on chalkboard

- Hypnotic dreaming

- Somatic or Affect Bridge

- Story without an ending (patient provides the ending)

- Disorientation in Time.

All the foregoing – all well and good, but ...

All of the above techniques are well and good; however, to develop your skills you need to move beyond pro forma induction, deepening, and story or technique. A psychologist once told me, "I think of what the client needs to hear in order to be well and I say it." To that end, what I do is *intersperse* my patter with suggestions aimed at the target: "You can do it ... you can let go ... you can be strong ... just let it be," or whatever *spontaneously* comes to mind. Techniques such as seeding or misspeak are important; however, to really develop your art you need to employ interspersal. Some therapists discuss a metaphor immediately afterward and some don't. Try both ways. Erickson strived for *integration* and you can do this by allowing a long silence at the end, before realerting: "Just appreciate the stillness for a few minutes ..." Ask them if they have any questions, spend some time on discussion, and emphasize the use of anchor and the importance of practicing relaxation, or using the CD you've made for them.

Two overarching principles guide me: (1) hypnosis as adjunct (i.e., it is seldom a complete treatment by itself, as clients are often taking medication, involved in talk therapy, support group, etc.) and (2) the words of Jeff Zeig: "Let the client's *response* be your guide, not the cleverness of the technique."

General approach

The first session I usually do no hypnosis. I take a history, listen closely to words and concepts that are important to them, and try to clarify a realistic goal. I want to assess control issues, negative stereotypes about hypnosis, and ferret out any magic bullet expectations. If they're at all reluctant to begin, I restrain, e.g., "This isn't for everybody. Think about it for a few weeks and then call me if you want to continue."

1. Induction, deepening, Three Lessons story; get them responding with finger signals, deep breath, head nod, etc.

- If at least some hypnotic phenomena are elicited:

  ▪ Next session: Balloons story

- Next session or two, depending on self-efficacy:

  ▪ ego-strengthening

- Following sessions:

  ▪ zero in on target using techniques mentioned above.

2. If no hypnotic phenomena are elicited first session:

- Next session:

  ▪ Consider directive induction or confusional induction.

3. If still no response:

- Stop hypnosis. Lack of response means either: (1) they want a magic bullet, or (2) their unconscious resistance is too strong. Spend your time on people who *do* respond, which is most others. Tell them their response indicates that they are among a small minority of the population who cannot benefit from hypnosis, and offer them other resources.

Glossary

absorption of attention Part of the induction phase and necessary for successful trance, the client's attention is focused on, for example, a story, a bodily sensation, a spot on the wall, or something else. Eye fixation, eye closure, diminished bodily movement, facial mask, and other signs may indicate a successful absorption of attention.

age progression Essentially the opposite of age regression – in trance clients are asked to imagine themselves in the future, perhaps feeling or behaving confident, strong, or in control. Therapists often tend to provide more structure for age progression than necessary, e.g., imagining pages of a calendar flipping forward, or imagining one's self in a time tunnel or similar device, when often all that is necessary is for the therapist to wait for a few seconds while clients take themselves to a future time. Typically clients are asked to signal, e.g., with a head nod "when you are there." The most famous example is Erickson's crystal ball technique. Also a hypnotic phenomenon.

age regression A technique useful in hypnosis for accessing resources during problem solving and other applications, age regression is a naturally occurring phenomenon whenever we have a memory or reminiscence. In hypnosis, age regression, like other therapeutic applications, follows the induction and deepening phases. It may be guided and structured, e.g., "Beginning now, I want you to ride a magic carpet back through time to age 15, and when you're there, in your mind, you may signal with your *yes* finger." If the therapist's intention is to implement the age regression, abreaction, and reframing technique to treat an incident of abuse at age 15, the therapist waits for the client to signal before continuing. Sometimes we don't have a target age and we "go fishing" for important data. To do this, a general and permissive age regression is usually sufficient, e.g., "Starting now, I want you to go back in time, in your own way, taking as much time as you need, to *any time* in the past that might be important for the problem at hand, and when you get there, let me know by nodding your head." When the client nods her head she may have gone back in time to ten minutes ago or ten years ago, and the only way we will know is by asking for a verbal report. Following the verbal report we will customarily ask her to continue her unconscious search until the process is completed. As with other techniques, we never want to surprise clients, and should tell them our intentions when setting the agenda during pre-trance discussion. Also, if relevant, it is important for us to remind clients that all memories, including those accessed through hypnosis may not be valid, as they could be distortion or fantasy. Also a hypnotic phenomenon.

age regression, abreaction, and reframing This eminently useful technique (Hammond, 1990) is very helpful for trauma, especially one-time incidents. After you explain the technique, proceed to induction and deepening and then age regress the client to the time of the event, induction and deepening are followed by age regression to the time of the event. We then ask them to abreact, or fully express, any feelings associated with the event, e.g., "Tell me now all the anger you have inside you ..." and do the same with fear, sadness, guilt, shame, or any other emotions. Have a box of tissues handy, as clients will typically cry, moan, blow their nose, or do other things associated with abreaction. When we feel there has been complete abreaction, we move on to reframing, e.g., "It is wonderful how you've released these pent-up feelings. I know that now, with the perspective of time and maturity you can move on and do well in your life." We can then seek unconscious commitment for same, e.g., "Let me ask a question of your unconscious mind … and that question is this, 'Are you willing to put this in the past, move on, and do well in the future?' You may answer with one of those fingers on your right hand."

amnesia Some practitioners believe that in some cases facilitating amnesia is necessary for later problem resolution, as amnesia allows unconscious processing to proceed without conscious interference. Amnesia can be suggested directly, e.g., "Beginning now, you may just forget anything from today that you wished to remember," or "The material today, will you remember to forget it, or just forget to remember?" A more indirect suggestion is, "Last night when I slept I had a dream, and when I woke up I could not remember the dream." Distraction may also facilitate amnesia, e.g., the client is realerted and immediately the therapist launches into an irrelevant story. Many clients will have amnesia for some portion of the trance experience even if it is not facilitated. Also, in many cases partial – not complete – amnesia may be a more realistic goal. Inducing amnesia may be helpful in treating episodic chronic pain.

amplifying the metaphor This technique is especially effective with anxiety and anger. In pre-trance discussion "the problem" is agreed upon, and following induction and deepening the therapist permissively elicits a symbol or metaphor (e.g., a color, an object, or anything concrete) for both the problem and the absence of the problem. Then, the problem is amplified, e.g., "Now, whatever symbol or representation you have for the problem, I want you to make it very strong, amplified. If it is the color red, intensify it, feel the red in all its brilliance beginning now, while I count to 3 … 1, 2, 3, and now, just let it go." Then, the same is done for the problem's absence while the therapist ties its absence to an anchor, e.g., "Make a circle with your right thumb and index finger and similarly make that symbol strong while I count, 1, 2, 3, very good, and just let that hand relax."

apposition of opposites Hypnotic language such as this is believed to be trance inducing. This technique juxtaposes opposites such as near–far, up–down, and inside–outside, e.g., "Another person one time noticed a *heaviness* developing in that *right* hand, while a *lightness* was detected in the *left* hand ..." Hypnotic language can be a major tool of the therapist in talk therapy as well as in hypnosis.

arm catalepsy Catalepsy means suspension of movement, and a cataleptic or rigid arm is employed in the arm catalepsy induction (Gafner and Benson, 2000), a highly directive but brief and effective means of inducing trance. It is contraindicated in people with cervical pain, peripheral neuropathy, and related conditions and some clients may appreciate a conversational or story induction instead.

authoritarian approach Such an approach in psychotherapy may involve telling clients in no uncertain terms what to do. A therapist who employs directive or authoritarian language in hypnosis may say, "You *will* now drop off into deep trance and you *will* lose your desire for cigarettes." Certainly some clients will respond better to this approach and I advocate a place for it in the therapist's toolbox. In a permissive and more indirect approach the operative word is *may* instead of *will*, e.g., "In a few moments you *may* begin to find yourself drifting off into trance, and I wonder when you will start to experience the pleasure of life without cigarettes."

automatic process This refers to mental functioning that is outside of a person's conscious awareness. Synonymous with unconscious process, a few of the techniques that access this process are metaphor, misspeak, and subtle vocal shift. Much of a person's mental functioning is unconscious and not governed by conscious intent and purpose. In this book, the unconscious is a vital target in hypnotherapy.

bind of comparable alternatives An example of hypnotic language, this technique appears to offer the client a choice between two or more alternatives, offering the illusion of choice, e.g., in hypnosis, "This session would you like to go into a light trance, a medium trance, or a deep trance?" Or in talk therapy, "The material we covered today might be pertinent to your personal life, useful at work, or maybe you can simply incorporate it into your overall experience."

confusion A broad category of techniques that are used to counter unconscious resistance, confusion typically distracts, interrupts, or overloads. In this book, confusional inductions are described. Another common confusional technique involves the non sequitur, e.g., during the induction or deepening, the therapist says, "At that store the shopping carts always stick together." The therapist pauses briefly while the conscious mind tries to make sense of this out-of-context statement, and then the therapist follows with a way out of the confusion, and in the desired direction, e.g., "And you can go deep." Confusion is indicated only when straightforward techniques have failed, and should always be used judiciously and respectfully.

contingent suggestion Also known as chaining, this type of suggestion connects a suggestion to an ongoing or inevitable behavior, thus making it more likely to be accepted, e.g., "... and as you begin to notice that familiar heaviness in your hand, you can let that comfort spread all throughout your body." A dentist who employs hypnosis may use contingent suggestion as a posthypnotic suggestion, e.g., "... and the next time you return here and settle into the chair, the moment I turn on this light you can begin to develop pleasant numbness in your mouth." (See also **leading**, **linking word**, and **truism**.)

debriefing A very important phase in the hypnotic process, this follows the realerting and is where the therapist ratifies hypnotic phenomena, answers questions, and elicits subjective experience. The therapist may learn important data, especially in the early sessions, e.g., "I couldn't hear you," or "That story you told me today about a lake, didn't you know I almost drowned in a lake?"

deepening Following the induction phase and before the therapy phase of hypnosis, trance is deepened in any variety of ways, often by counting down from 10 to 1. In this book, for instructional purposes I break down a hypnosis session into pre-trance discussion, induction, deepening, therapy phase, realerting, and debriefing. Many who practice hypnosis roll these phases into one, or use no formal deepening.

displacement Used in pain management, the locus of pain is imaginally displaced to another part of the body, or outside the body, e.g., "The discomfort in your knee, why should one knee hog all the pain ... you can allow 30% of it to be shared by the little finger on your left hand ..." The client typically will continue to experience the sensation, but hopefully with less pain in the target area. It is important for the therapist to think pattern interruption and diminution of the pain rather than the elimination of it.

dissociation Dissociation is a hallmark feature of trance as well as an excellent ratifier or convincer of trance. The more clients experience dissociation, e.g., hands or feet separated from the body, the richer the hypnotic experience. Encouraging dissociation is recommended even with clients who experience dissociation pathologically, e.g., with post-traumatic stress disorder (PTSD), and the strategy may be explained to such clients as capitalizing on a natural ability. The same is true for other pathological features, such as psychological numbness and spacing out. Employing dissociative language, e.g., *that* hand instead of *your* hand, facilitates dissociation.

ego-strengthening Self-efficacy or ego-strength is defined as believing that one's behavior will lead to successful outcomes. To many, ego-strength is also seen as the ability to cope with environmental demands. This book describes two types of hypnotic ego-strengthening, short burst and metaphorical. The author posits that major therapeutic gains may be made with hypnotic ego-strengthening for anxiety, mood, and chronic pain disorders even without employing corrective or abreactive measures. Hypnotic ego-strengthening techniques are explained to the client as "a mental building up," something appreciated by persons with chronic problems. Of course, consciously directed ego-strengthening, such as coping skills training and other skill building and similar measures, should be applied as well.

embedded suggestion An exquisitely useful tool in hypnosis, this is also referred to as embedded command or embedded meaning. An inward focus can be encouraged, e.g., "Going *inside* can be very *in*teresting ... *in* there where you have your imag*in*ation, *in*tuition ..." A psychologist in Phoenix was working with a client on weight loss and wanted to encourage walking. He mentioned another client who bought a *wok* ... and *wokking* became his preferred manner of food preparation. The client lost 80 pounds, kept it off, and is still walking.

eye closure This can be suggested by phrasing such as, "Your eyes may blink and those eyelids might feel heavy, and those eyes can close whenever you wish ..." Eye closure can also be seeded through rehearsal prior to the induction, e.g., "Close your eyes very briefly while I count to 3 ... now how did that feel?" However, some clients, especially those with PTSD, may not wish to close their eyes during hypnosis. It is best for the therapist to not push eye closure if a client is reluctant to do so, as sufficient depth may occur by fostering absorption of attention in eye fixation alone.

eye fixation For clients who fear loss of control, the therapist may ask them to focus their gaze on a spot of their choice, e.g., on the wall or the back of the hand. Most clients eventually become comfortable enough to close their eyes.

fluff Therapists often think that every word in an induction or story should be purposeful or didactic. However, meaningless, meandering detail, or fluff, may deepen absorption and serve to increase receptivity to key suggestions. Also, a few well-placed suggestions amidst the fluff may be very effective.

hidden observer This is a phenomenon experienced by nearly everyone in trance and it is good to point it out to the client, e.g., "You have your conscious mind, your unconscious mind, and your hidden observer, the part of you that observes what's going on." People's hidden observer usually diminishes after the first session or two; however, if it remains active it may impede the client's letting go. Then, a confusional induction may be indicated.

hypnotic language Hypnotic language is thought to fascinate, connect with the unconscious, and to foster absorption. In this book, bind of comparable alternatives, implication, power words, and other concepts are subsumed under hypnotic language.

hypnotic phenomena This term refers to catalepsy, dissociation, time distortion, amnesia, automatic writing and drawing, arm levitation, anesthesia, positive and negative hallucination, and other phenomena that are both naturally occurring phenomena as well as phenomena that may occur in trance. Inductions in this book contain many suggestions for hypnotic phenomena and once experienced by the client they should be ratified or reinforced.

ideomotor finger signal To avoid the client's becoming a passive recipient, and in order to learn important data, it is important for the client to communicate during hypnosis. This "dance," or back-and-forth communication can occur via a head nod, verbal report, or finger signal. The author typically asks clients to put their hands out on their lap so they can be observed, and then, in trance, the therapist elicits preferences for fingers – usually on the preferred or dominant hand – that can signify *yes, no,* and *I don't know/not ready to answer yet.* Then, say, you've processed a particular symptom and want to know if the client is ready to let go of it, you ask, "Now, I want to ask a question of your unconscious mind, and the question is this, 'Are you ready to put X behind you and move on?' Taking as much time as you need, you may answer with one of your fingers." It is believed that a mere twitch of the finger represents a true unconscious communication (and a response that is available on the finger before it is available on the tongue), whereas a deliberate lifting of the finger is a conscious response. Sometimes a finger signal is not evident and during debriefing the client says, for example, "I thought my *yes* finger moved."

implication With implication, the operative word is *when*, not *if*, e.g., "I wonder *when* you'll notice heaviness in your hands?" or "Which one of your hands feels heavier?" In accessing unconscious resources, the therapist may say, "*When* the back part of your mind has selected some strength or resource that served you well in the past, your *yes* finger can move all by itself."

indirection Indirection generally refers to an unconsciously directed approach. To tell a client an anecdote or story about someone else who successfully managed her anger is an indirect suggestion, while a directive approach for the same problem would involve straightforward instruction. The higher the reactance or resistance, the more indirection is indicated.

induction The phase of hypnosis where trance is induced. As described in this book, the other parts of the process include pre-trance discussion, (induction), deepening, therapy, realerting, and debriefing.

instigative anecdote or story Useful for clients who are "stuck," this metaphorical approach is designed to be self-referenced by the client in order to stimulate unconscious problem solving.

interspersal First described by Milton Erickson, this invaluable indirect technique involves interspersing the therapist's hypnotic patter – or induction, deepening, or story – with key suggestions, such as "Just let go," or "You can do it." If this random insertion is preceded by a pause, attention is riveted. If the client is analytical, it is useful to lead away after the suggestion, e.g., "*Just let go* – and I can't stop thinking of that barking dog yesterday." Then, the suggestion may percolate in the unconscious without analysis. The author usually informs clients that he may be saying things that don't make sense in order to "get in underneath the radar." The therapist's approach is always framed as helping.

law of parsimony This "law" holds that the therapist should do only what is necessary to achieve the desired effect. For a client who is experienced with trancework, a lengthy induction may not be necessary, and all that need be done is, "Just sit back now, let those eyes gently close, settle into that chair and taking as much time as you need, let a deep trance develop all on its own … and when you're sufficiently deep in order to do the work we need to do today, your *yes* finger will rise."

lead away This is a confusion technique that is used to distract the conscious mind from a preceding suggestion by saying something irrelevant, e.g., *"You can overcome this problem – and let me tell you how those shopping carts stuck together at the grocery store."* Such techniques are useful with clients who show unconscious resistance.

leading Pacing and leading are important in communication to show understanding. The word *and* has been called the most important word in psychotherapy because it links and leads to suggestions or directives. So, in discussion following hypnosis, we might say, "I know how nervous you feel in social situations, *and* I think it's important for you to regularly practice your anchor that we covered in hypnosis today."

linking word We may offer the client a series of truisms followed by *and* before a suggestion. Similarly, "You exhale *and* you can feel tension leaving your body." (See also **contingent suggestion, leading,** and **truisms**.)

metaphor We listen for metaphors offered by clients so they can be utilized in therapy. "There is a wall around me" is a therapeutic invitation to "loosen the mortar between the bricks, knock a hole in the wall, lower the wall for one hour in the morning," or any variety of pattern interruption. The most common types of metaphors in hypnosis are story and anecdote.

misspeak This elegant indirect technique should be used sparsely to be most effective in communicating a suggestion to the unconscious. For example, "The man changed his behavior across the *board/border* up in Canada." The therapist appears to misspeak, the first word is the suggestion and the second word serves to lead away. The author may prepare misspeak for clients by asking himself the question, "What do they need to hear in order to be well?"

naturalistic trance states Discussion prior to hypnosis should ask when a client normally drifts off or becomes pleasantly absorbed in something like a movie or song. Many experience "highway hypnosis" while driving. By comparing hypnosis in the office to naturally occurring behavior there may be less fear of loss of control.

non sequitur Used for distraction or interruption, this is a brief, out-of-context phrase used to interrupt conscious mental sets. When the therapist offers a non sequitur, the client strives to make sense of it, and the therapist offers a way out – and in the desired direction, e.g., "Why did it rain last week?" followed by a suggestion such as, "You can go deep." Employed in short-burst ego-strengthening.

not knowing/not doing Actually a suggestion for restraint, clients find this device quite liberating in that it fosters unconscious responsiveness and dissipates conscious effort. This suggestion tends to free up the untrained trance subject who is trying very hard to "get it right." It is also thought to assist in discharging anxiety or resistance. In an induction the author usually adds, "There's absolutely nothing at all that you need to know, or do, or think about, or change, in fact, all you really need to do is just sit there and breathe. There's nowhere you need to be, nothing to accomplish, and you don't even have to listen to the words, which can drift in and drift out."

pattern interruption First described by Milton Erickson and further developed by Cade and O'Hanlon (1993), among others, this elegant and wide-ranging technique is a major tool in the toolbox of practitioners of strategic and other brief therapies. Clients often come to us and desire to *eliminate* their problem, and when therapists approach the goal in this way both parties often end up disappointed. It is eminently easier – and more realistic – to aim instead for *altering* one aspect of the problem which in turn often results in problem resolution. To effect this, we work with the client to alter the intensity, frequency, duration, location, or some other aspect of the problem. For example, for a father and daughter who typically argue in the kitchen in the morning, the therapist asks them, "I want you to indulge me in a little experiment, which is this: I would like you to limit your arguing to only Monday, Wednesday, and Friday in the living room. Are you willing to do that?" Pattern interruption is a wonderful technique for virtually any individual problem as well as relational problems. Rationales presented to clients are either an experiment, or to try and bring the problem under voluntary control.

pause Believed to be a form of indirect suggestion, the therapist pauses for a couple of seconds during, say, an induction or story. A pause causes the listener to begin an unconscious search, and clients may at that moment be receptive to suggestion. For example, in a story, "He was searching for something and in the afternoon he found it when (pause) *he saw a flash of light.*" Or, used after a suggestion, "He made a significant discovery (pause) which *came as a total surprise.*" The author also uses pause as a suggestion, though less indirectly: "During the session you may hear a pause (pause), or a period of silence, and I don't mean the paws on a cat or dog, and you may use these times to let your experience deepen."

permissive suggestion Many clients respond better if given a wide range of choice: "You may begin to notice sensations, feelings, experiences, or even something else peculiar or curious in your hands, feet, or elsewhere in your body." This may also be expressed with less verbosity: "Beginning now and taking as much time as you need, let yourself experience anything at all in your body or your mind."

perturbation The author's simple rule of thumb: when stuck, perturb. This helps clients to break out of rigid points of view or dysfunctional behavior. Your target for perturbation is always the unconscious, and instigative anecdotes or stories are a major way to perturb. If you, as a therapist, are stuck, try reading an instigative story or several anecdotes to yourself, move on to doing something else, let them percolate in your unconscious for a few days, and then see what spontaneously might spring to mind.

posthypnotic suggestion This is a suggestion presented in trance for a behavior to occur outside of trance. For example, "When you return here next time and sit down again in that chair, the comfort of the chair will be a signal for you to begin to drift off." The author employs this suggestion for subsequent sessions, as above, to trigger relaxation outside the office by use of the anchor, and in unconscious problem solving.

power words Certain words in hypnosis may enhance the trance process, as they are believed to access the unconscious, or at least induce a sense of wonderment or curiosity. Examples are story, imagine, wonder, notice, curious, explore, intriguing, appreciate, and interesting. Authors such as Gilligan (1987) and others frequently combine notice and appreciate, e.g., "When you *notice* that familiar sensation in your hand, you may begin to *appreciate* the pleasantness of trance." In this book, power words are subsumed under hypnotic language.

pre-trancework discussion This is the initial part of a hypnosis session where the therapist "checks in" with the client and sets the agenda.

question Deceivingly simple yet quite elegant, a direct question asked during trance can rivet attention, stimulate associations, and facilitate responsiveness. During the induction, we may ask, " … a highly curious sensation in one hand, do you notice it yet?" The author often reaches for: "What is beginning to percolate *now* in your unconscious mind?" When the therapist senses resistance, which is usually *un*conscious, such a question may bring it to the fore, where it can be discussed and problem solved once the client is realerted.

reactance Resistance is to reactance as tide is to ocean, or guilt is to shame – a behavior or attitude that may be part of a larger whole. A reactant individual fears loss of control and in the author's experience most clients who have high reactance will not accept a referral for hypnosis.

realerting This is a part of the hypnosis session that follows the therapy component. The author typically uses, "Beginning now, I'm going to count from 1 up to 5 and by the time I reach 5 you can resume your alert, waking state, as if waking up from a nice, pleasant, refreshing nap, (increased volume), 1, 2, …"

Many clients are not eager for trance to end, or may require a few minutes to realert, so be patient.

reframe Reframing is a vital technique in most methods of psychotherapy, as the therapist's conveyance of new information provides the client with a new understanding or appreciation of a behavior or attitude. The client may see something in a new light, or be given hope, after a problem is given a positive connotation. "Just coming to this first session has to take some *courage* and that tells me there is hope," the author is prone to say. Virtually any problem or attitude can be reframed with a value thought dear to the client: closeness, duty, protectiveness, love, strength, loyalty, and caring are but a few. Therapists should be judicious with their reframes, as most clients are accustomed to hearing politicians and others say things like, "This is both a challenge and an opportunity," about some dreadful problem. In talk therapy, we can tell immediately from non-verbals whether the reframe is accepted. In hypnosis, a reframe is most commonly effected via metaphor, e.g., a story or anecdote about *someone else* who gains a different understanding or appreciation.

repetition Anything that is important, such as a suggestion or directive, should be repeated – but not too much. The author may repeat "breathing in comfort and relaxation" in an induction, and suggestions may also be repeated differently, e.g., "A cool, refreshing breath can be most enjoyable."

resistance Many times what we perceive as resistance to hypnosis may simply be anxiety about a new experience. "I don't want to go into trance" is probably high reactance and, of course, hypnosis will not be pursued further. However, "I *want* to go into trance but just *can't*" is likely unconscious resistance, which may be an indication for a confusional induction, but which also may be successfully discharged by permissive suggestions, a suggestion covering all possibilities, not knowing/not doing, metaphor, and similar devices. Resistance can also be discharged by having clients change chairs (so the resistance is left in the first chair), or by asking them questions which must be answered by "no," e.g., (in Tucson) "It's not hot out today, is it?" Most clients are keenly aware of their

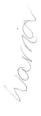

resistance, which will abate through reassurance, or as they become more comfortable with the process.

restraint Let's say you've conducted a couple of sessions with a person and he doesn't practice using his anchor or listen to the CD made for him. The author usually restrains, or holds them back from moving ahead, e.g., "Change may mean uncertainty ... we may be moving too fast ... you may not be ready for this ... or, perhaps you should think about it for a few weeks before we reschedule." When the author has clients who are anxious or resistant, for the first session or two he typically begins an induction, realerts, asks them how they're doing, then resumes the induction. If necessary, he will realert and reinduce more than once. Holding back something pleasant or potentially helpful builds responsiveness and enhances client control.

seeding A suggestion may be more successful if it has been seeded beforehand. To do this, the target suggestion is mentioned (seeded) early on, and later, by mentioning the target again, the "seed" is activated. If the problem is anxiety and in the therapy component the author's target is slowing down, he may say to the client, "The traffic on the freeway sure was *slow* this morning." To seed this non-verbally, the author may *slowly* get up from his chair to retrieve a pen, and *slowly* return to his chair. Later on, when *slowing down* is mentioned in a story, the seed is activated. Seeding is akin to foreshadowing in literature when, say, dark, foreboding clouds presage tragedy. It is also similar to priming in social psychology. In one experiment to influence subjects' choice of laundry detergent, guess which product was chosen by those who were primed with the word pair ocean/moon? Yes, it was Tide. This unconsciously directed technique is well worth the little preparation required ahead of time.

short burst As used in this book, short burst is employed in ego-strengthening. A non sequitur is offered ... and followed shortly by a suggestion, e.g., "Why do dogs bark? ... You can go deep." When not used with a confusional suggestion such a non sequitur, it is the same as interspersal. In addition to short burst the author employs metaphorical ego-strengthening.

story The story is a vital metaphorical approach and a prim ary means for offering suggestions in hypnosis. As an indirect technique, a story goes in "underneath the radar," meaning that it cannot be defended against or consciously analyzed. Essential to a story is embedded suggestion.

suggestion covering all possibilities When the therapist mentions several suggestions, the likelihood of the client's accepting one or more may be more likely, e.g., "As a person goes deeper into trance various sensations may begin to develop in the hands or feet ... a tingling or numbness in one hand or that hand on the other side ... coolness or warmth in one or both feet ... maybe a heaviness up here, a lightness down there, or some other intriguing sensation in the extremities or elsewhere in the body." The author often reaches for metaphor in this situation: "One woman one time, she detected, just noticed, an itching in her right earlobe, and in the left ..."

therapy component As described in this book, a phase of the hypnosis session that may consist of a story or stories, age progression or age regression, unconscious exploration or problem solving, or a highly structured technique such as amplifying the metaphor. Some practitioners have no clear phases.

time distortion An important hypnotic phenomena that is important to elicit and ratify, especially early on. In this book suggestions for time distortion are embedded in many of the inductions. Time expansion and time contraction are contained in, "In trance, time may seem to speed up or slow down." After realerting the person in the first session it may be relevant to ask, "How much time do you think passed here today?" All hypnotic phenomena experienced by the client should be reinforced.

truism This is an undeniable statement of fact. A series of truisms leads to a "yes-set" and acceptance of suggestions. In talk therapy, the author may say, "Okay, we've met three times now, all sessions were at 3 p.m. We've explored your anger and feelings about your ex-wife ... *and* between now and next time I'd like you to do X." In hypnosis, he may say, "Coming in here today on this rainy day, having to wait five minutes extra in the waiting room, and finally coming in here, sitting down there, you know and I know that today especially you can drift off into the deepest of trances."

unconscious mind Milton Erickson and others believed that much of a person's mental functioning is governed not by conscious intention and deliberate choice, but by features that operate outside of conscious awareness and control. Findings in psychological research have confirmed this (Bargh and Chartrand, 1999). Some clients may mean unconscious when they say subconscious or back part of the mind. The author may describe it to clients as "that part of you that takes over when you're dreaming, or daydreaming."

unconscious problem solving The hypnotherapist may instigate problem solving on an unconscious level with a variety of techniques including directives or other suggestions to the unconscious, with instigative anecdotes or stories, or with, for example, a permissive suggestion that is tagged to a behavior known to occur in the natural environment. With the latter, say the therapist knows that the client drives by Broadway and Fifth nearly every day. The therapist offers the suggestion that "you will learn something important to help you with your problem" when he passes through that intersection, followed with a suggestion for amnesia. Next session the client returns with a new resource but has no awareness of how or why. This technique works best with clients in whom amnesia is easily fostered.

unconscious process In psychology literature this is more often referred to as automatic process, or that which lies outside of one's immediate awareness. Techniques such as metaphor, pause, and misspeak are believed to access this process.

unconsciously directed therapy A cornerstone of this approach in hypnosis or psychotherapy is metaphor and story, whose purpose is to influence the unconscious mind. Cognitive behavioral therapy is primarily concerned with conscious mechanisms, whereas other approaches – like Gestalt, psychodrama, or psychodynamic therapy – employ techniques directed at both the conscious and unconscious mind.

utilization If they give you lemons, make lemonade. That is an example of utilization in daily life, as is this: the U.S. war in Vietnam left thousands of bomb craters, which many people converted to duck ponds after the war. In psychotherapy, or hypnosis, the client's behavior, however problematic, is accepted and utilized, or employed, to transform the problem. A treatment philosophy more than a mere technique, "utilization dictates that whatever the patient/family brings to the sessions can be harnessed to effect a psychotherapeutic result" (Zeig and Geary, 2000). This is a fundamental principle of Ericksonian therapy, as interpretation is to psychoanalysis, or desensitization to behavior therapy. For a client who is very rigid, the therapist may reframe the behavior as steadfast purpose and say, "Let's start to make some purposeful changes with which you can feel comfortable." For hypervigilant clients who are reluctant to close their eyes, the therapist may encourage attentional absorption with eye fixation on a spot on the wall. Erickson had a family therapy case where the husband's complaint was his wife's secretive drinking, while the wife complained about her husband's spending time with his "dirty old magazines." The couple had an old camper in the driveway that they had not used for many years, a symbol of their unhappiness. They had formerly used the camper to go fishing, an activity they both detested. Erickson got their agreement for directives involving the wife's "hiding your whiskey bottle where he'll never find it." She soon grew tired of the game. The directive to go fishing followed, and the couple began to enjoy camping once again, began to appreciate each other's company, and learned that they no longer needed either the drinking or the old magazines (Zeig and Geary, 2000).

References

Anabar, R. D. and Hummell, K. E. (2005). Teamwork approach to clinical hypnosis at a pediatric pulmonary center. *American Journal of Clinical Hypnosis*, 48 (1), 45–49.

Araoz, D. L. (1998/1982). *The New Hypnosis in Sex Therapy.* Northvale, NJ: Jason Aronson.

Araoz, D. L. (2005). Hypnosis in human sexuality problems. *American Journal of Clinical Hypnosis*, 47 (4), 229–242.

Barber, J. (1996). *Hypnosis and Suggestion in the Treatment of Pain.* New York: W.W. Norton and Co.

Bargh, J. A. and Chartrand, T. L. (1999). The unbearable automaticity of being. *American Psychologist*, 54 (7), 462–479.

Blanchard, E. B. (2005). A critical review of cognitive, behavioral, and cognitive-behavioral therapies for irritable bowel syndrome. *Journal of Cognitive Psychotherapy: An International Quarterly*, 19 (2), 101–123.

Brickman, H. (2000). *The Thin Book: Hypnotherapy Trance Scripts for Weight Management*. Phoenix, AZ: Zeig, Tucker, and Theisen.

Brown, D. and Fromm, E. (1987). *Hypnosis and Behavioral Medicine*. Hillsdale, NJ: Erlbaum.

Cade, B. and O'Hanlon, B. (1993). *A Brief Guide to Brief Therapy*. New York: W.W. Norton and Co.

Childs, C. (2001). Below the rim. *Arizona Highways*, 79 (12), 20–31.

Dolan, Y. (1991). *Resolving Sexual Abuse*. New York: W.W. Norton and Co. – cited p. 50.

Dossey, L. (1999). Foreword. In R. Temes (ed.), *Medical Hypnosis* (pp. vii–viii). New York: Churchill Livingstone.

Edgette, J. H. and Edgette, J. S. (1995). *The Handbook of Hypnotic Phenomena in Psychotherapy*. New York: Brunner/Mazel.

Elkins, G., Marcus, J., Palamara, L., and Stearns, V. (2004). Can hypnosis reduce hot flashes in breast cancer survivors? A literature review. *American Journal of Clinical Hypnosis*, 47 (1), 29–42.

Ewin, D. (1992). Hypnotherapy for warts: 41 consecutive cases and 33 cures. *American Journal of Clinical Hypnosis*, 35 (1), 1–10.

Fass, R. (forthcoming). Hypnotherapy in the treatment of noncardiac chest pain of presumed esophageal origin: A randomized clinical trial.

Feldman, J. B. (2004). The neurobiology of pain, affect and hypnosis. *American Journal of Clinical Hypnosis*, 46 (3), 187–200.

Feldman, J. B. (2009). Expanding hypnotic pain management to the affective dimension of pain. *American Journal of Clinical Hypnosis*, 51 (3), 235–254.

Gafner, G. (2004). *Clinical Applications of Hypnosis*. New York: W.W. Norton and Co.

Gafner, G. (2006). *More Hypnotic Inductions*. New York: W.W. Norton and Co.

Gafner, G. and Benson, S. (2000). *Handbook of Hypnotic Inductions*. New York: W.W. Norton and Co.

Gafner, G. and Benson, S. (2001). Indirect ego-strengthening in treating PTSD in immigrants from Central America. *Contemporary Hypnosis*, 18 (3), 135–144.

Gafner, G. and Benson, S. (2003). *Hypnotic Techniques*. New York: W. W. Norton abd Co.

Geary, B. (1999). *Personal Communication*. Phoenix, A.Z.: Zeig, Tucker, and Theisen.

Gilligan, S. G. (1987). *Therapeutic Trances: The Cooperation Principle in Ericksonian Hypnotherapy*. New York; Brunner/Mazel.

Golden, W. L. (2007). Cognitive-behavioral hypnotherapy in the treatment of irritable-bowel syndrome-induced agoraphobia. *International Journal of Clinical and Experimental Hypnosis*, 55 (2), 131–146.

Goldstein, R. H. (2005). Successful repeated hypnotic treatment of warts in the same individual: A case report. *American Journal of Clinical Hypnosis*, 47 (4), 259–264.

Gonsalkorale, W. M. (2006). Gut-directed hypnotherapy: The Manchester approach for treatment of irritable bowel syndrome. *International Journal of Clinical and Experimental Hypnosis*, 54 (1), 27–50.

Gordon, C. M. and Gruzelier, J. (2003). Self-hypnosis and osteo pathic soft tissue manipulation with a ballet dancer. *Contemporary Hypnosis*, 20 (4), 209–214.

Green, J., Barabasz, A., Barrett, D., and Montgomery, G. (2005). The 2003 APA Division 30 definition of hypnosis. *American Journal of Clinical Hypnosis*, 48 (2–3), 89.

Hammond, D. C. (1990). *Handbook of Hypnotic Suggestions and Metaphors*. New York: W.W. Norton and Co.

Hammond, D. C. (2008). Hypnosis as sole anesthesia for major surgeries: Historical and contemporary perspectives. *American Journal of Clinical Hypnosis*, 51 (2), 101–121.

Iglesias, A. (2004). Hypnosis and existential psychotherapy with end-stage terminally ill patients. *American Journal of Clinical Hypnosis*, 46 (3), 201–213.

Iglesias, Alex, and Iglesias, Adam (2005). Awake-alert hypnosis in the treatment of panic disorder: A case report. *American Journal of Clinical Hypnosis*, 47 (4), 249–258.

Jensen, M. (2008). The neurophysiology of pain perception and hypnotic analgesia: Implications for clinical practice. *American Journal of Clinical Hypnosis*, 51 (2), 123–148.

Kingsbury, S. J. (1988). Hypnosis in the treatment of post-traumatic stress disorder: An isomorphic intervention. *American Journal of Clinical Hypnosis*, 31 (2), 81–90.

Kirsch, I., Montgomery, G., and Sapirstein, G. (1995). Hypnosis as an adjunct to cognitive-behavioral psychother apy: A meta-analysis. *Journal of Consulting and Clinical Psychology*, 63 (2), 214–220.

Kleibeuker, J. H. and Thijs, J. C. (2004). Functional dyspepsia. *Current Opinion in Gastroenterology*, 20 (6), 546–550.

Lankton, S. (2007). Psychotherapeutic intervention for numerous and large viral warts with adjunctive hypnosis: A case study. *American Journal of Clinical Hypnosis*, 49 (3), 211–218.

Lankton, S. R. and Lankton, C. H. (1983). *The Answer Within: A Clinical Framework of Ericksonian Hypnotherapy.* New York: Brunner / Mazel.

Liquid Mind (1994). Music CD. Sausalito, CA: Real Music.

Lynn, S. J. and Hallquist, M. N. (2004). Toward a scientifically based understanding of Milton H. Erickson's strategies and tactics: Hypnosis, response sets and common factors in psychotherapy. *Contemporary Hypnosis*, 21 (2), 63–78.

Marquis, A. L. (2006). Higher Learning: The science behind how trees get tall ... and what keeps them from growing taller. *National Parks Magazine,* Spring, pp. 14-18.

Martensen, R. L. (1997). Hypnotism's medical heyday. *Journal of the American Medical Association*, 277 (8), 611.

Mills, J. C. and Crowley, R. J. (1986). *Therapeutic Metaphors for Children and the Child Within.* New York: Brunner / Mazel.

Nichols, T. (2000). *Glen Canyon: Images of a Lost World.* Alburquerque, N.M.: University of New Mexico Press.

Olness, K. (1980). Imagery (self-hypnosis) as adjunct therapy in childhood cancer: Clinical experience with 25 patients. *American Journal of Pediatric Hematology / Oncology*, 3, 313–321.

Patterson, D. R, Hoffman, H. G., Weichamn, S. A., Jensen, M. P., and Sharar, S. R. (2004). Optimizing control of pain from severe burns: A literature review. *American Journal of Clinical Hypnosis*, 47 (1), 43–54.

Pekala, R. J., Maurer, R., Kumar, V. K., Elliott, N. C., Masten, E., Moon, E., and Salinger, M. (2004). Self-hypnosis relapse prevention training with chronic drug/alcohol users: Effects on self-esteem, affect and relapse. *American Journal of Clinical Hypnosis*, 46 (4), 281–297.

Poon, M. W. (2009). Hypnosis for complex trauma survivors: Four case studies. *American Journal of Clinical Hypnosis*, 51 (3), 263–271.

Potter, G. (2004). Intensive therapy: Utilizing hypnosis in the treatment of substance abuse disorders. *American Journal of Clinical Hypnosis*, 47 (1), 21–28.

Powers, P. (2006). The practice of slowing down. *All Things Considered*. National Public Radio, April 3, 2006.

Prochaska, J. O., DiClemente, C. C., and Norcross, J. C. (1992). In search of how people change. *American Psychologist*, 47, 1102–1114.

Rosen, S. (1982). *My Voice Will Go with You: The Teaching Tales of Milton H. Erickson*. New York: W.W. Norton and Co.

Rossi, E. L. (1980). *Collected Papers of Milton H. Erickson (Vols 1–4)*. New York: Irvington.

Rossi, E. L. (2003). Gene expression, neurogenesis, and healing: Psychosocial genomics of therapeutic hypnosis. *American Journal of Clinical Hypnosis*, 45 (3), 197–216.

Rossi, E. L. (2006). *A Discourse with Our Genes*. Phoenix, AZ: Zeig, Tucker, and Theisen.

Rossi, E. L. and Cheek, D. B. (1988). *Mind–Body Therapy: Methods of Ideodynamic Healing in Hypnosis.* New York: W.W. Norton and Co.

Samuels, N. (2005). Integration of hypnosis with acupuncture: Possible benefits and case examples. *American Journal of Clinical Hypnosis,* 47 (4), 243–248.

Schoenberger, N. E. (2000). Research on hypnosis as an adjunct to cognitive-behavioural therapy. *International Journal of Clinical and Experimental Hypnosis,* 48 (2), 154-169.

Shenefelt, P. D. (2004). Using hypnosis to facilitate resolution of psychogenic excoriations in acne excoriee. *American Journal of Clinical Hypnosis,* 46 (3), 239–245.

Shoham-Salomon, V. and Rosenthal, R. (1987). Paradoxical interventions: A meta-analysis. *Journal of Consulting and Clinical Psychology,* 55, 22–27.

Spanos, N. P., Williams, V., and Gwynn, M. I. (1990). Effects of hypnotic, placebo, and salicylic acid treatments on wart regression. *Psychosomatic Medicine,* 52 (1), 109–114.

Sperr, E. and Hyer, L. (1994). Stress management in the care of PTSD. In L. Hyer (ed.), *Trauma Victim* (pp. 587–632). Muncie, IN: Accelerated Development.

Stiefel, J. R. (2006). The clocks in the collection. *Magazine of Antiques,* Aug., 88–93.

Tan, G., Hammond, D. C., and Gurrala, J. (2005). Hypnosis and irritable bowel syndrome: A review of efficacy and mechanism of action. *American Journal of Clinical Hypnosis,* 47 (3), 161–178.

Taylor, E. E., Read, N. W., and Hills, H. M. (2004). Combined group cognitive-behaviour therapy and hypnotherapy in the management of the irritable bowel syndrome: The feasibility of clinical provision. *Behavioural and Cognitive Psychotherapy, 32,* 99–106.

VandeVusse, L., Irland, J., Berner, M. A., Fuller, S., and Adams, D. (2007). Hypnosis for childbirth: A retrospective comparative analysis of outcomes in one obstetrician's practice. *American Journal of Clinical Hypnosis,* 50 (2), 109–119.

Wain, H. J. (2004). Reflections on hypnotizability and its impact on successful surgical hypnosis: A sole anesthetic for septoplasy. *American Journal of Clinical Hypnosis,* 46 (4), 313–321.

Wallas, L. (1985). *Stories for the Third Ear.* New York: W.W. Norton and Co.

Walsh, B. J. (2003). Utilization sobriety: Brief, individualized substance abuse treatment employing ideomotor questioning. *American Journal of Clinical Hypnosis,* 45 (3), 217–224.

Whorwell, P. J. (2008). Hypnotherapy for irritable bowel syndrome: The response of colonic and noncolonic symptoms. *Journal of Psychosomatic Research,* 64, 621–623.

Winerman, L. (2006). From the stage to the lab. *Monitor on Psychology,* 37 (3), 26–27.

Wood, G. J., Bughi, S., Morrison, J., Tanavoli, Sara., Tanavoli, Sohrab, Zadeh, H. H. (2003). Hypnosis, differential expression of cytokines by T-cell subsets, and the hypothalamo-pituitary-adrenal axis. *American Journal of Clinical Hypnosis,* 45 (3), 179–193.

Yapko, M. D. (1992). *Hypnosis and the Treatment of Depressions: Strategies for Change.* New York: Brunner/Mazel.

Yapko, M. D. (2001). *Treating Depression with Hypnosis: Integrating Cognitive-Behavioral and Strategic Approaches.* New York: Brunner/Routledge.

Yapko, M. D. (2005–2006). Some comments regarding the Division 30 definition of hypnosis. *American Journal of Clinical Hypnosis*, 48 (2–3), 107–110.

Yexley, M. J. (2007). Treating postpartum depression with hypnosis: Addressing specific symptoms presented by the client. *American Journal of Clinical Hypnosis*, 49 (3), 219–223.

Young, C. A. (2007). Unpublished manuscript.

Young, J. V. (1990). *Kokopelli: Casanova of the Cliff Dwellers and the Hunchbacked Flute Player*. Palmer Lake, CO: Filter Press.

Zeig, J. K. and Geary, B. B. (eds) (2000). *The Letters of Milton H. Erickson*. Phoenix, AZ: Zeig, Tucker, and Theisen.

Zlotogorski, Z. and Anixter, W. L. (1983). The use of hypnosis in the treatment of reflux esophagitis: A case report. *American Journal of Clinical Hypnosis*, 25 (4), 232–234.

Further Reading

For Further Study

I regularly read the *American Journal of Clinical Hypnosis* (www. asch.net); *Contemporary Hypnosis*, a publication of the British Society of Clinical & Academic Hypnosis (www.bsech.com); and the *International Journal of Clinical and Experimental Hypnosis* (www.ijech.com). Another fine journal is the *Australian Journal of Clinical and Experimental Hypnosis* (www.ozhypnosis. com.au). Additional resources are the British Society of Medical and Dental Hypnosis (www.bsech.com) and the Royal Society of Medicine, Section for Hypnosis and Psychosomatic Medicine (*www.rsm.ac.uk/academ/smth_p.php*). Some newsletters, such as those of The American Society of Clinical Hypnosis (www.asch.net), The International Society of Hypnosis (www.ish-web.org), The Milton H. Erickson Foundation (www.erickson-foundation.org). can help you keep abreast of developments in the field.

I continue to learn a great deal from many books on hypnosis, Some of these are listed below:

Hypnosis: Questions and Answers, by Bernie Zilbergeld, M. Gerald Edelstien, and Dan Araoz

The Letters of Milton H, Erickson, by Jeff Zeig and Brent Geary

Brief Therapy: Myths, Methods, and Metaphors, by Jeffrey Zeig and Stephen Gilligan, Eds.

Ericksonian Methods: The Essence of the Story, by Jeffrey Zeig, Ed.

Ericksonian Psychotherapy, vols. I and II, by Jeff Zeig, Ed.

Treating Depression with Hypnosis and *Trancework: An Introduction to the Practice of Clinical Hypnosis,* by Michael Yapko

Resolving Sexual Abuse, by Yvonne Dolan

Handbook of Hypnotic Suggestions and Metaphors, by D. C. Hammond

The Psychobiology of Mind-Body Healing, by Ernest Rossi

Mind-Body Therapy, by Ernest Rossi and David Cheek

Therapeutic Metaphors for Children and the Child Within, by Joyce Mills and Richard Crowley

Therapeutic Trances and *The Legacy of Milton H. Erickson: Selected Papers of Stephen Gilligan* by Stephen Gilligan

In Search of Solutions, by Bill O'Hanlon and Michelle Wiener-Davis

A Brief Guide to Brief Therapy, by Bill O'Hanlon and Brian Carle

Assembling Ericksonian Therapy, by Stephen Lankton

The Answer Within: A Clinical Framework of Ericksonian Hypnotherapy, by Stephen Lankton and Carol Lankton

Tales of Enchantment: Goal-Oriented Metaphors for Adults and Children in Therapy, by Stephen Lankton and Carol Lankton

and, last but not least, the valuable works of Milton H. Erickson, two of which are *Hypnotic Realities*, by Milton Erickson, Ernest Rossi, and Sheila Rossi. and *The Collected Papers of Milton H. Erickson on Hypnosis, vols. I-IV*, by Ernest Rossi, Ed.

Hypnosis Organizations

American Society of Clinical Hypnosis

  www.asch.net

Australian Society of Hypnosis

  www.ozhypnosis.com.au

British Society of Clinical & Academic Hypnosis

  www.bsach.com

International Society of Hypnosis

  www.ish-web.org

Milton H. Erickson Foundation

  www.erickson-foundation.org

New Zealand Society of Hypnosis

  www.nzsh.org/nz

Royal Society of Medicine, Section for Hypnosis and Psychosomatic Medicine

www.rsm.ac.uk/academ/smth_p.php

Society of Clinical and Experiemental Hypnosis

www.sceh.us

Index

abreaction 95, 98, 106,

acceptance 22, 44, 48, 51, 93, 120

age progression 20, 22, 55, 95, 98, 101, 102, 105, 120

age regression 3, 20, 22, 76, 95, 98, 100, 101, 102, 105, 106, 120

amnesia 4, 35, 83, 100, 107, 112, 121

amplifying the metaphor 15, 95, 98, 107, 120

anchor 51, 74, 95, 103, 107, 114, 117, 119

anecdotes 47, 64, 95, 99, 116, 121

anxiety 5, 14, 22-26, 95, 98, 107, 110, 115, 118, 119

apposition of opposites 32, 33, 52, 54, 55, 63, 96, 108

arm catalepsy 108

attention, absorption of 105, 111

attentional absorption 122

authoritarian approach 4, 108

automatic process 14, 108, 121

Benson, S. 20, 22, 23, 48, 89, 98, 99, 101, 108, 125

bind of comparable alternatives 108, 112

breathing 19, 32, 65, 85

catalepsy 4, 25, 32, 33, 52, 72, 73, 98, 108

children 98, 127, 134, 135

cognitive behavioural therapy (CBT) 12, 15, 17, 21, 24, 25, 47, 94, 100, 121, 123, 125, 126, 129, 130, 131

commitment 51, 107

communication (in trance) 96, 112

confidence 15, 42

confusion 86, 89, 90, 109, 114

confusional inductions 4, 81-90, 104, 109, 111, 118

conscious mind 51, 85, 109, 111, 114

contingent suggestion 109, 114

contrasts 63

control issues 11, 12, 103

crystal ball technique 105

debriefing 13, 36, 42, 48, 56, 73, 109, 112, 113

deepening 36, 41, 46, 48, 51, 56, 57, 65, 70, 73, 76, 79, 86, 100, 103, 104, 106, 107, 109, 110, 113

dentistry 19

displacement 101, 103, 110

dissociation 4, 10, 22, 24, 32, 34, 35, 36, 54, 55, 56, 70, 98, 101, 110, 112

dissociative language 54, 56, 110

distraction 79, 89, 101, 107, 115